P9-DEQ-363

REIKI
MASTERY

REIKI
MASTERY

FOR SECOND DEGREE, ADVANCED, AND REIKI MASTERS

DAVID VENNELLS

BOOKS

Winchester, UK
New York, USA

Copyright © 2004 O Books
46A West Street, Alresford, Hants SO24 9AU, U.K.
Tel: +44 (0) 1962 736880 Fax: +44 (0) 1962 736881
E-mail: office@johnhunt-publishing.com
www.johnhunt-publishing.com
www.o-books.net

U.S. office:
240 West 35th Street, Suite 500
New York, NY10001
E-mail: obooks@aol.com

Text: © 2004 David Vennells
Design: Jim Weaver Design

ISBN 1 903816 70 X

All rights reserved. Except for brief quotations in critical articles or
reviews, no part of this book may be reproduced in any manner without
prior written permission from the publishers.

The rights of David Vennells as author have been asserted in
accordance with the Copyright, Designs and Patents Act 1988.

A CIP catalogue record for this book is available
from the British Library.

Printed in Singapore by Tien Wah Press (Pte) Ltd.

ACKNOWLEDGEMENTS

Many thanks to everyone who has helped in the
preparation and completion of this book.

Illustrations of Medicine Buddha on page vii and
Wheel of Life on page 33 reproduced with kind permission
of Tharpa Publications, www.tharpa.com.

For information about other books by the same author
visit www.healingbooks.co.uk

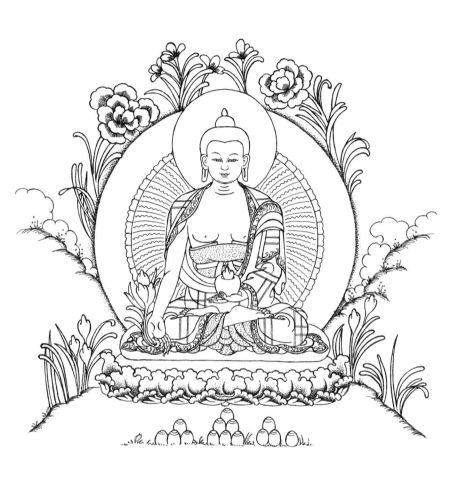

Medicine Buddha

CONTENTS

INTRODUCTION

The response to my first book on Reiki, *Reiki For Beginners* (Llewellyn Books) was very encouraging. I really enjoyed writing it and learned so much in the process that I soon found myself planning a book on the "higher" levels of Reiki. Many readers of *Reiki For Beginners* have said that the Buddhist content helped to answer many of their questions about Reiki, how to develop a special relationship with Reiki and how we can use Reiki to best effect either as a healing therapy for body and mind or as tool for spiritual and personal growth. Advanced practitioners and Masters also mentioned that a book with a similar approach to "Higher" Reiki would be very helpful.

For a while I was unsure about beginning such a book; it seemed like a big task and I felt overwhelmed at the prospect of crossing uncharted waters. It is a cliché that "the longest journeys begin with one step" but it is true. Making the first step was the hardest but once the wheels were in motion the main part of the book developed naturally. As with the first book it has been a wonderful project to be involved in; I feel I have relearned Reiki. I hope after reading it that you feel the same and if necessary return to it whenever you need clarification on some issue or simply to "realign" your path.

I have been very fortunate to receive my First, Second, and Master Degree Reiki training from three different Masters. This is not always recommended as a relationship with a one good Master can be a very valuable aid to your growth. This gives you time to really get to know them and for them to get to know you and this mutual knowledge can be most valuable when learning the advanced levels of Reiki as your Master can answer your questions and point you in the right direction based on the personal relationship you have developed.

However, in my case this was not to be and now I can see why! Each of my Masters taught Reiki in different ways, some of these differences were obvious and some quite subtle. All three were excellent Masters. Their commitment and devotion to their vocation is unquestionable. What is interesting is that despite the apparent differences in the style of teaching the Reiki was the same! The same very special, timeless, loving, forgiving, protecting presence was there in abundance in all three classes.

So I learned from this that I have to find my own way of living and representing Reiki, not to slavishly follow others but simply to take from others what I think is right for me and most importantly to let Reiki guide me in the direction that is most natural and that is most beneficial to others. So I hope this is how you will use this book. Much of what I have written is not gospel. You can decide through trial and error what is right for you and discard the rest or just put it on hold.

Anything that I have included from a Buddhist perspective is as close to the way it was presented to me as possible. If you feel uncomfortable with any of the Buddhist content just put these ideas on hold for a while and come back to them at a later date if you wish. I am still a beginner and have no deep experience of the real essence of Buddhism so if you are interested in this path it is really important that you follow up with further reading of authentic Buddhist texts like those mentioned in Appendix 5. If you want to find or help establish a local Buddhist meditation class look at the information given in Appendix 4.

The three Reiki Masters that I trained with very kindly allowed me to make many notes during my Reiki training and it is these notes that form the main part of the framework of this book. I am not normally one for making notes in classes and usually just like to sit back and soak things up. But even from the beginning of my first degree training I felt compelled to take detailed notes and it is only now, years later, that I am beginning to realize how valuable they are. Without them I could not have written this book and shared much of the knowledge that has made and is making my life with Reiki so enjoyable and meaningful.

Also, I must say that the greater part of this book has been made possible only because of the kindness of my own spiritual guide, who has written many books and given many teachings without which my life with Reiki, although still special, would have been without any clear focus or meaning. The teachings that he gives are without parallel and it is only possible for me to pass on a little of what they mean and how they can help us realize the true meaning of our life.

I hope you find this book very helpful and interesting,

Wishing You Good Health and Great Happiness.

PREFACE

When I began my Reiki training I never thought that I would become a teacher of Reiki and I think most Reiki "Masters" felt the same at the beginning of their Reiki Life. I suppose life is like that generally anyway. Things never quite work out as we expect. Sometimes they work out better than we expect and sometimes worse. So this tells us that planning our future in detail is a waste of time and that making the most of what we have while we have it is good life management. No matter what provisions we make for our future, with regard to money, career, relationships, etc., we will not be able to prevent difficulties of one kind or another arising. We all know that no matter how hard we try we cannot avoid such difficulties as ageing, sickness, and death – these are inevitable sufferings. At present this potential for suffering is in our very nature as human beings, if we had a choice no one would choose to grow old and die.

This might seem like a bleak outlook and a strange introduction to a Reiki book that should be encouraging a positive perspective on life! However, facing the facts of life is the fuel for a swift, enjoyable, and clear spiritual path toward inner and outer healing. Some people might have the impression that Reiki, especially the advanced levels of practice, is about beautiful, spiritual, other-worldly experiences as we activate our upper chakras and contact our higher self on another plain of existence. If this is what you want, no problem, Reiki can take you there. But if you want it for the wrong reasons it can be just another selfish high, just another distraction, just another way of avoiding the real issues.

Advanced Reiki, if practiced correctly, is really about facing yourself, looking within, moving down through the chakras and dealing with your "stuff." We can do this for ourselves, for our own benefit, which is fine and very worthy. Or simply by adapting or changing our mental intention or motivation we can do this for others. This reversal of motivation is very special, very powerful and the consequences or effects of such altruistic mental intentions are phenomenal. We can even adopt this intention every time we read this book simply by thinking "may every living being benefit from my actions of reading this book and studying these techniques." This is such a simple but powerful spiritual practice and we can apply it to so many areas of our life and we will look at this fascinating way of living in more detail later.

Dealing with our own "stuff" by reducing selfishness, impatience, ignorance, developing special minds like love, compassion, empathy, patience, and wisdom may seem like hard work or not as interesting as "out of body" experiences or other spiritual highs. However, in reality the special spiritual experiences that many people long for are ironically a natural byproduct of this path. Simply seeking spiritual highs for our own benefit can actually cause more problems in the long run.

If we consider the great spiritual teachers like Jesus, Buddha, Krishna, Mohammed and even more recent spiritual leaders like Gandhi and the Dalai Lama all these special beings teach the path of compassion, the path of empathy and regard for the welfare of others. Disciples of Jesus know that he even gave his own life to benefit others. We cannot conceive what kind of special spiritual realizations these beings experienced. They were only able to achieve these through developing their compassion and wisdom, which brought them very close to their spiritual father or mother, maker or source. Perhaps they became inseparable, the same nature as the "source," simply through their continuous effort (through meditation and prayer) to develop the same good qualities and by becoming a pure channel for that sublime consciousness to benefit others.

So it is with Reiki, if we develop the motivation of studying and practicing the advanced levels of Reiki so that we can help others by developing the precious minds of compassion and wisdom then our path can be swift, smooth, and blissful!

DR. USUI'S MEMORIAL INSCRIPTION

The following translation can be found at
www.threshold.ca/reiki/usui_memorial_translation.html
and is reproduced here with kind permission of Richard Rivard.

Translation of the Usui Memorial
at Saihoji Temple, Tokyo Japan

© Universal Copyright 1998–2003 Emiko Arai and Richard Rivard
Please feel free to share this with others others – as is, with no changes

Since a friend in Japan sent us pictures of the Usui memorial in the spring of 1996, we had been wanting to put this web page up. Many other projects got in the way, and we didn't get a good close-up of the monument until our friend Shiya Fleming brought back some good photos in July, 1997. Emiko and I spent several days going through several old dictionaries she had, and I was very happy at the end to compensate her for her part in the process. Finally, I felt we completed enough to present this to others.

This is a fairly literal translation of the Usui memorial, as we wanted you, the reader, to get as close a rendition to plain English as possible, without any paraphrasing. This allows you to decide how you would rephrase sentences and paragraphs. There are a few phrases that we haven't translated yet.

All comments in (brackets) are either our translations of previous kanji (in quotations), or our explanation of previous words. Please note: there are no periods or paragraphs on the original, so we have added these in to make it easier to read. Also, as in all translations, we had several choices of words for each kanji, and tried to pick what we felt best. Our thanks to Melissa Riggall and Miyuki Arasawa for their corrections offered.

Although this location does contain the remains of Usui Sensei's wife – Sadako; son – Fuji; and daughter – Toshiko, it only has a part of Sensei's remains. The Saihoji site was set up 11 months after Sensei's death and is not his original resting place. In fact, Sensei's living students (there are several) say he was a Tendai Buddhist all his life, while the Saihoji temple is a Jodo Shu (Pure Land) Buddhist temple. There is a small private shrine elsewhere in Tokyo that hold the original remains, as well as the original Usui Affirmations (Precepts) on a wall hanging, and the original large photo portrait of Sensei taken by Dr. Hayashi.

Please share this information with all, but we ask you to leave this portion and copyright with it. For pictures and location of the memorial, please visit my Saihoji Temple pages.

(I would like to express my gratitude to all those who have offered changes and corrections to the translation)

TRANSLATION BEGINS

"Reihou Chouso Usui Sensei Kudoko No Hi"
Memorial of Reiki Founder Usui Sensei's Benevolence

(The top of the memorial reads, from right to left: "Reihou" – spiritual method, Reiki method; "Chouso" – founder; "Usui"; "Sensei" – teacher; "Kudoku" – benevolence, a various (pious) deed; "no Hi" – of memorial, a tombstone, a monument – this is also what the first line in the main text says).

It is called 'toku' that people experience by culture and training, and 'koh' that people practice teaching and the way to save people. ('koh' + 'toku'= 'kudoku; Kou = distinguished service, honor, credit, achievement; Toku = a virtue, morality)

Only the person who has high virtue and does good deeds can be called a great founder and leader. From ancient times, among wise men, philosophers, geniuses and ? (a phrases that means – very straight and having the right kind of integrity), the founders of a new teaching or new religion are like that. We could say that Usui Sensei was one of them.

Usui "Sensei" (literally "he who comes before", thus teacher, or respected person) newly started the method that would change mind and body for better by using universal power. People hearing of his reputation and wanting to learn the method, or who wanted to have the therapy, gathered around from all over. It was truly prosperous. (by "therapy" is meant the Usui Reiki Ryoho – Usui ancestral remedy – of his Usui-Do teachings, including the 5 principles.)

Sensei's common name is Mikao and other name was Gyoho (perhaps his spiritual name). He was born in the Taniai-mura (village)in the Yamagata district of Gifu prefecture (Taniai is now part of Miyama Village). His ancestor's name is Tsunetane Chiba (a very famous Samurai who had played an active part as a military commander between the end of Heian Period and the beginning of Kamakura Period (1180-1230). However this person is now known not to be Usui's anscestor. See the notes at the end on the Usui family Ancestors.) His father's name was Uzaemon (this was his popular name; his given name was Taneuji). His mother's maiden name was Kawai.

Sensei was born in the first year of the Keio period, called Keio Gunnen (1865), on August 15th. From what is known, he was a talented and hard working student. His ability was far superior. After he grew up, he traveled to Europe, America and China to study (yes, it actually says that!). He wanted to be a success in life, but couldn't achieve it; often he was unlucky and in need. But he didn't give up and he disciplined himself to study more and more.

One day he went to Kuramayama to start an asceticism (it says "shyu gyo" – a very strict process of spiritual training using meditation and fasting.) On the beginning of the 21st day, suddenly he felt one large Reiki over his head and he comprehended the truth. At that moment he got Reiki "Ryoho" (This term originally meant ancestral remedy or therapy) (Note: this experience on Kuramayama seems to be unknow by Sensei's surviving students, so he may not have shared this with many.) When he first tried this on himself, then tried this on his family, good results manifested instantly. Sensei said that it is much better to share this pleasure with the public at large than to keep this knowledge to our family (it was customary to keep such knowledge in the family to increase their power). So he moved his residence to Harajuku, Aoyama, Tokyo (this is next to the Meiji Outer Gardens and the huge Aoyama Cemetery.) There he founded "Gakkai" (a learning society) to teach and practice Reiki Ryoho in April of the 11th year of the Taisho period (1922) (Actually at this time, according to his student Tenon-in (who in 2003 is 106), he was teaching his spiritual method simply called "his method" or Usui-Do.") Many people came from far and wide and asked for the guidance and therapy, and even lined up outside of the building. (This is another fact that has not been verified by Usui Sensei's surviving students. His senior living student explained that from 1920 Sensei taught a spiritual system called Usui-Do, from which his students created Usui Reiki Ryoho in 1925.)

September of the twelfth year of the Taisho period (1923), there were many injured and sick people all over Tokyo because of the Kanto earthquake and fire. Sensei felt deep anxiety. Everyday he went around in the city to treat them. We could not count how many people were treated and saved by him. During this emergency situation, his relief activity was that of reaching out his hands of love to suffering people. His relief activity was generally like that. (Mr. Hiroshi Doi was told that Sensei would actually lay on the ground and give Reiki from his hands and feet to at least 4 people at time)

After that, his learning place became too small. In February of the 14th year of the Taisho period (1925), he built and moved to a new one (a dojo or training hall) outside Tokyo in Nakano. (Nakano is now part of Tokyo.) Because his fame had risen still more, he was invited to many places in Japan, often. In answering those requests, he went to Kure, then to Hiroshima, to Saga and reached Fukuyama. (Fukuyama was also the location of Sensei's creditors – his final trip was mainly to meet with them). It was during his stay in Fukuyama that he unexpectedly got sick and died. He was 62 years old. (In Western terms, Sensei was 60 – born August 15, 1865; died March 9, 1926 as per his grave marker; however, in old Japan, you are "1" when born and turn another year older at the start of the new year). His wife was from Suzuki family; her name was Sadako. They had a son and a daughter. The son's name was Fuji who carried on the Usui family (meaning the property, business, family name, etc. Born in 1908 or 1909, at the time of his father's death Fuji was 19 in Japanese years. We learned that Fuji may ahve taught Reiki in Taniai village. According to the Usui family grave stone, the daughter's name was Toshiko, and she died in September 23, 1935 at the age of 22 in Japanese years -21 in Western years. Sensei also taught his wife's niece who was a Tendai Buddhist Nun. As of this writing (2003) she is still alive – approximately 108).

Sensei was very mild, gentle and humble by nature. He was physically big and strong yet he kept smiling all the time. However, when something happened, he prepared towards a solution with firmness and patience. He had many talents. He liked to read, and his knowledge was very deep of history, biographies, medicine, theological books like Buddhism Kyoten (Buddhist bible) and bibles (scriptures), psychology, jinsen no jitsu (god hermit technique), the science of direction, ju jitsu (he also learned Judo from Jigoro Kanao, accoring to Tenon-in), incantations (the "spiritual way of removing sickness and evil from the body"), the science of divination, physiognomy (face reading) and the I Ching. I think that Sensei's training in these, and the culture which was based on this knowledge and experience, led to the key to perceiving Reiho (short for "Reiki Ryoho"). Everybody would agree with me. (The origins of the Usui-Do system are now known to be from Taoism brought to Japan from China, probably around the 5th century.)

Looking back, the main purpose of Reiho was not only to heal diseases, but also to have right mind and healthy body so that people would enjoy and experience happiness in life. Therefore when it comes to teaching, first let the student understand well the Meiji Emperor's admonitory, then in the morning and in the evening let them chant and have in mind the five precepts which are:

First we say, today don't get angry.
Secondly we say, don't worry.
Third we say, be thankful.
Fourth we say, endeavor your work.
Fifth we say, be kind to people.

(My friend Emiko Arai was very firm about the above wording.)

This is truly a very important admonitory. This is the same way wisemen and saints disciplined themselves since ancient times. Sensei named these the "secret methods of inviting happiness", "the spiritual medicine of many diseases" to clarify his purpose to teach. Moreover, his intention was that a teaching method should be as simple as possible and not difficult to understand. Every morning and every evening, sit still in silence with your hands in prayer (gassho) and chant the affirmations, then a pure and healthy mind would be nurtured. It was the true meaning of this to practice this in daily life, using it. (i.e. put it into practical use) This is the reason why Reiho became so popular. (see the Usui Precepts for more on this.)

Recently the world condition has been in transition. There is not little change in people's thought. (i.e. it's changing a lot) Fortunately, if Reiho can be spread throughout the world, it must not be a little help (i.e. it's a big help) for people who have a confused mind or who do not have morality. Surely Reiho is not only for healing chronic diseases and bad habits.

The number of the students of Sensei's teaching reaches over 2,000 people already (This number may also include the students'

students). Among them senior students who remained in Tokyo are carrying on Sensei's learning place and the others in different provinces also are trying to spread Reiki as much as possible. (Dr. Hayashi took title to the dojo in November, 1926 and together with Admiral Taketomi and Admiral Ushida, re-located it to his clinic in Shinano Machi in 1926, and ran it as a hospice.) Although Sensei died, Reiho has to be spread and to be known by many people in the long future. Aha! What a great thing that Sensei has done to have shared this Reiho, which he perceived himself, to the people unsparingly.

Now many students converged at this time and decided to build this memorial at Saihoji Temple in the Toyotama district (local boundaries have changed and the Saihoji temple has been in Nakano district (1986) and is now in Suginami district) to make clear his benevolence and to spread Reiho to the people in the future. I was asked to write these words. Because I deeply appreciate his work and also I was moved by those thinking to be honored to be a student of Sensei, I accepted this work instead of refusing to do so. I would sincerely hope that people would not forget looking up to Usui Sensei with respect . (The location of the burial plot and memorial may have been the work of the Admirals and the URR Gakkai. Usui Sensei was confimed by his liviing students Tenon-in and Suzuki-sensei to have been a devout Tendai until his death. Yet the Saihoi temple is a Pure Land sect or Jodo Shu Buddhist temple.)

Edited by "ju-san-i" ("subordinate third rank, the Junior Third Court (Rank) – an honorary title), Doctor of Literature, Masayuki Okada.

Written (brush strokes) by Navy Rear Admiral, "ju-san-i kun-san-tou ko-yon-kyu"("subordinate third rank, the Junior Third Court (Rank), 3rd order of merit, 4th class of service" – again, an honorary title) Juzaburo Ushida (also pronounced Gyuda).

Second Year of Showa (1927), February

I

─ O R I G I N A L   R E I K I ─

The Story of Dr. Usui Revisited

Most Reiki people know that Reiki came to the West from Japan and that the founder of Reiki was Dr. Mikao Usui. Dr. Usui died on 9 March 1926 and by that time had established a large Reiki community in Japan. His successor was a Mr. Ushida and after his death there were four more presidents until the present leader or figurehead of the Japanese Reiki tradition Mr. Kondo, who took over from a Ms. Koyama in 1998.

Dr. Usui's memorial inscription – which appears on the preceding pages – is a special link to "Original Reiki" and it is worth reading regularly until we begin to grasp the essence of what it represents. It is an excellent reminder of how we should approach our daily practice and helps us to value and appreciate Dr. Usui's extraordinary legacy.

Reiki came to the West via Reiki Master Hawayo Takata who practiced mainly in Hawaii. Toward the end of her life she taught a handful of Masters who began to introduce Reiki more widely in the USA from where it spread to Europe and the rest of the world. Mrs. Takata's teacher or Master was Dr. Chujiro Hayashi who was one of Dr. Usui's students.

There will probably be conflicting thoughts and feelings in the Western Reiki community for some time regarding the issues of whether the concept of a Western Grand Master is valid. Also whether the various "new" types of Reiki are acceptable and helpful. There are no clear answers to these issues that will satisfy all of us. However, this might not be a bad thing if we regard it as an opportunity to practice tolerance. Reiki moves in mysterious ways, perhaps the Reiki that we practice, whatever its form or origin is just right for us at present. However, it is worth considering that the more we "add" to the original Reiki format the further we are from original Reiki as taught by Dr. Usui.

Whatever our lineage or techniques we all have one spiritual Reiki Father, Dr. Usui, and this can never change. Dr. Usui was the focal point at which Reiki entered our dimension. He is our living link to the purity and clarity of "original Reiki." We might think that he is gone from this world and that it is too late to be close to him or to develop a meaningful relationship with him, but this is not so.

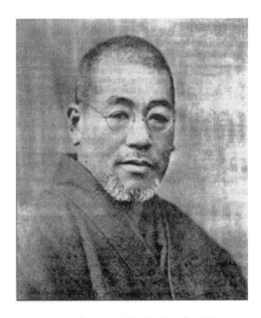

Dr. Mikao Usui 'The Father of Reiki'

We do not have to be physically near someone to feel close to them. In fact we can be physically very close to someone yet feel very distant. So it is with our relationship with Dr. Usui – we may not be able to talk directly with him but we can definitely feel and develop a very close connection with him. If we didn't already have a close karmic connection with him we would not have found Reiki. So it will probably not be too difficult for us to develop this relationship further.

If we have faith that Dr. Usui is the Father of Reiki, that he was or is a living example of the essence of the Reiki path then that is what he will be for us. If we think that Dr. Usui is a dead Japanese man who lived a long time ago in a world very different from our own then that is what he will be for us. We can choose to impute whatever qualities we wish on him. But if we feel close to him and try to develop a special affection or respect for him then we can gain great benefit in our Reiki practice.

It is not wise to put him on a pedestal though, or to see him as some other-worldly superior being, as this again creates a barrier or distance; just view him as a close friend or relation. Someone who is there to help you, someone who understands, who has been through the same things that you are experiencing, and has great empathy, wisdom, and a sense of humor. If you feel comfortable you can view Reiki and Dr. Usui as the same nature. If we already have a strong faith/religion and a spiritual guide like Jesus or Buddha or a spiritual teacher still alive in a human form then we can regard them as our Reiki guide/master. If we feel uncomfortable with the idea of having a guide or teacher then we can just focus on Reiki and our own inner wisdom. Ultimately it is our own inner wisdom that is the supreme spiritual guide but while we are developing this quality it is really helpful to have a friend to guide us.

So not everyone will feel comfortable with this approach but it is just an idea that you might find helpful if you feel your Reiki practice needs a lift or you want to take things to another level. It also helps us all, whatever our religion, lineage, or form of practice, to focus on our similarities as Reiki children with one farther/mother just "appearing" in different aspects as Jesus, Buddha, Dr. Usui, and so on. There is a benevolent omniscient force in this universe that is constantly with us and quietly encouraging us in the right direction. Reiki, especially above first degree, is about "facing the mirror," the "inner mirror" of our own mind. Presently this mirror is covered in dirt and the images we begin to see are distorted by the accumulated confusion gathered over countless lifetimes. As we progress with our spiritual practice we can clean away the layers of misconception that color the way we view ourselves, others, and the world around us. Eventually the mirror will become clean and we will directly realize our true nature as the mirror itself! We will look more closely at this idea later.

Higher Reiki

We may wonder why there are different levels of Reiki and why we have to learn Reiki in stages. Each stage is complete in itself so we can stop at whatever level we feel comfortable with and we do not have to continue training above first degree. In fact to continue to second degree and above just for the sake of completing these is a waste of time. Some people have chosen to complete all the levels of training and have even become Reiki Masters in a very short time. This may "work" in some cases and a very few people might be ready for such a leap in the type of Life Force Energy they carry. However, experience shows that we get the most from Reiki by taking the time to really integrate each level of training with our life. It is really important to value Reiki (not necessarily in a financial sense) to give ourselves time and space to let Reiki come into our lives and work on us.

In fact there are many first degree practitioners who are actually more spiritually advanced than some "Masters." It is very easy to become a Reiki Master nowadays, at least by name. But it is not so easy to become a sincere Reiki practitioner.

The term "Master" is actually misleading, "teacher" might be a more appropriate term. The word Master suggests mastery, meaning complete experiential and intellectual understanding, someone who has mastered their chosen vocation. Who can master Reiki?! A true Reiki Master is really a Reiki Servant and, even more difficult to swallow, a servant to those who need Reiki. In these days of personal empowerment and glorification of fame and power it is not very cool to be a servant. Yet these are the kind of humble qualities we need if we want to get close to Reiki and away from our ego, the source of most of our problems. The higher levels of Reiki can really empower us in this journey toward real inner peace and freedom from problems. But if we learn the higher levels as an ego trip we will encounter problems sooner or later.

Many Masters recommend at least 3–6 months between each level of Reiki training. If we can it is better to wait until we are "called." We will know in our hearts when this happens, and it is usually when our ego becomes less interested in advanced Reiki for the kudos it might hold for us. The best way of overcoming our ego toward the higher levels is to think that we are doing this for others and that by moving closer to the heart of Reiki our ego will naturally lose power and we will find more contentment and peace of mind. Often our ego will not like this and begins to think of lots of reasons not to do it. That is often the best time to do it, as that is when we may make the greatest progress. However, it is always a middle way and we do not want to cause ourselves mental strain by over-challenging ourselves as this can be another way that our ego hijacks our spiritual progression.

There is no problem with staying at first or second degree level. There is so much we can do with Reiki at any level that we don't necessarily need to continue the training. What really matters is the skill and motivation with which we use Reiki. Having the certificates and titles is of little benefit if we are not sincerely using Reiki with a good heart and wise mind and we can learn how to do this whatever our level of practice.

Western Reiki

Reiki in the West has four well-known levels. First and second degree, advanced and Master level. Originally there were just three as advanced level was not separate from Masters. Advanced Reiki is really Master level for those who have no intention to teach but would like to carry the Master energy and work on themselves at that level.

These four levels are well established in the Western tradition and seem to work very well. We know now that traditional Japanese Reiki is different in that seven levels of Reiki are taught. The Japanese equivalent of first degree is actually split in four levels and the Reiki Master has to be sure that the student has mastered each level before the next is taught. Whereas first degree in the West is taught over one weekend, in Japan the four levels could take months to learn and included the studying and recitation of spiritual poetry, the Reiki principles, breathing exercises, lectures on Reiki from the teacher, and the well known Reiki empowerments.

The fifth level is very similar to the Western second degree and is separated in to a mental and emotional healing section, using symbols, and a distant healing section. The sixth level is quite rare and not many people are fortunate to receive this; the people at this level have the opportunity to become a Reiki teacher's assistant and to practice Reiki professionally. This ensures that the people who practice Reiki professionally on the general public are genuine, sincere, and highly trained individuals.

Finally the seventh level is Reiki teacher or Master. Even fewer people attain this level and the level of commitment to Reiki and to the welfare of Reiki students and patients is total.

So if you know a little of the current state of Western Reiki you will see that there are some glaring differences with "original Reiki"! At some point someone, maybe Mrs. Takata or Dr. Hayashi, made changes to the practice for the benefit of those they were teaching. Actually they made it simpler, which is what we like in the West. We have a fast pace of life and we are more impatient nowadays and many people are attracted to Reiki now because it is quick and easy to learn the basics, which is great; if the original format had been retained Reiki might not have spread so far so quickly.

Actually the form of Reiki has changed as well. In first degree we have 12 hand positions and these are taught so that the student can give a "full" Reiki treatment. But these are not taught in traditional Japanese Reiki where the hands are allowed much more free movement following the healer's intuition as in spiritual healing. Also there are techniques like gently blowing on areas of the body, stroking the air near the body, actually stroking the body, and even just looking at the body, i.e. using the eyes to transmit Reiki.

The 12 well-known hand positions are very useful for beginners as they cover the whole body and are easy to learn. But we don't have to keep to this form; we can experiment with friends and work out the techniques that work best for us. One of the good things about using regular hand positions is that it ensures a continuous flow of energy and allows the patient to relax. If we are blowing and stroking and waving our hands in the air this can be quite disturbing and worrying for someone with no experience of healing techniques. It can also be a distraction for us and entertaining for our ego! So we need to keep things simple and clear but also be open to new ideas and not be afraid to trust our intuition. If in the middle of a treatment we feel the need to gently blow on an area to clear stagnant energy or to place our hands in an unconventional position then go with it, although be sure that the patient feels comfortable with your actions first.

It is possible that much of Western Reiki will revert to the original Japanese form. Although Reiki is now so widespread outside Japan in different forms that it is unlikely that one form will prevail. In fact there are a few different offshoots from traditional Japanese Reiki and many Japanese people practice Reiki that they have learnt in the West! There are even Western Reiki Masters teaching in Japan!

The great thing about all this is that, as mentioned earlier, the

Reiki is still the same, still as effective, whatever form it is taught in. Surely Reiki "knew" how things would develop and may have actually caused or created things to work out as they have. Perhaps Western Reiki is not really missing anything; maybe it is fine as it is. As long as we have received the Reiki empowerments and basic techniques from a sincere teacher who received it from their teacher who can trace a clear lineage back to Dr. Usui then we have Reiki with us. We don't need to go to Japan to find Reiki, it is right here with us. We just have to continue developing our use and experience of it.

Reiki in the Buddhist tradition

Some Reiki practitioners are now aware that Dr. Usui was a Buddhist. However, there must now be far more non-Buddhist Reiki practitioners worldwide than actual Buddhist practitioners. So this should reassure us that Reiki is not Buddhist and we do not have to compromise any of our beliefs to benefit from Reiki. It doesn't matter how we try to explain or characterize Reiki it still works! No doubt Dr. Usui taught Reiki to his students within the framework of Buddhism: he must have explained the laws of karma and the importance of using Reiki with a good motivation. But there are many Masters today who teach Reiki within the framework of Christianity, and other religions.

This book tends to explain things from a Buddhist perspective in the hope that it will give Western practitioners deeper insight into the way Reiki was originally taught. Although Buddha's teachings are over two thousand years old they are still completely relevant to modern life. We can see that the external world has changed dramatically since the time of Buddha; however, our internal world is still very similar. The problems that we encounter in day-to-day life are identical to those of our ancestors. Problems with relationships, money, work, possessions, status, health, family are just the same issues people had to deal with thousands of years ago. Also, minds like impatience, greed, depression, anger, jealousy, discontentment again are exactly the same inner problems that our ancestors had to work with! The wisdom that Buddha teaches is the direct antidote to such problems, it offers practical and lasting solutions and is completely relevant in the modern world.

So it is hoped that the reader will find information from the Buddhist tradition to be enjoyable and interesting but not too challenging or threatening. Like most Buddhists Dr. Usui was not out to convert others or promote his religion; his wish was simply to help others find some lasting peace of mind and freedom from difficulties. So if you find that you cannot accept some of the material contained in this book, no problem, just use what helps you to develop a closer relationship with Reiki and put the rest on hold.

2

The Five Reiki Principles – Traditional Western Version
Just for today, do not worry.
Just for today, do not anger.
Honor your parents, teachers, and elders.
Earn your living honestly, (and put effort in to spiritual practice).
Show gratitude to every living thing.

One of the main differences between Japanese and Western Reiki is that we, in the West, tend to place less emphasis on Reiki as a spiritual practice. Many people regard and use Reiki as a simple healing technique for body and mind. Although many people also regard Reiki as a path to personal or inner growth not many regard it principally as a spiritual path. The byproducts of this path are the physical and mental healing aspects but in the West we tend to focus on this aspect because this is what we feel most comfortable with. So in some ways Reiki has been diluted or watered down to suit the Western mind.

This attitude is not necessarily wrong, if this is as far as we want to take Reiki then of course that is fine. There is no doubt that if we use Reiki purely as a healing technique then, although we will receive certain spiritual benefits, we will mainly just receive healing for body and mind. If we regard and learn to use Reiki as a spiritual path or as an aid to our existing spiritual path, then in time we will receive the greatest benefits that Reiki can give. We know that Dr. Usui was a practicing Buddhist and that he taught Reiki within the context of his understanding of this spiritual path. We also know that he thought it very important to regard Reiki as a spiritual practice to gain the most from it. Nowadays some Reiki practitioners find that after a few months or years of practice they are not deriving the same level of physical and mental benefit from their Reiki treatments as they used to, although the people that they treat still receive great results. A few people even say that the power of Western Reiki now is diminishing because it has become so separated from the original tradition. If this were true then all Reiki practitioners would be experiencing the same problem but this is plainly not the case as many continue to enjoy an increasingly powerful and profound level of experience as the years and months go by. So what is happening here?

The power of Reiki cannot change from its own side. Its nature is complete perfection, compassion, and wisdom, unchanging, timeless, transcendent, and beyond normal comprehension. The only thing that can change is our attitude, outlook, and relationship with Reiki. As time goes by if our view of Reiki gradually becomes ordinary then our experience and relationship with Reiki will also become ordinary. Like any relationship we need to work at it from time to time. From our side we need to make a little effort to progress without always relying on Reiki to do things for us.

Actually we usually just need to remember that "the path," whatever name we give it, is one of personal transformation and realization and not one of arranging everything in the external world to suit us.

Power without wisdom

Reiki in the West is often hailed as an empowering energy that we can use to create or attract and maintain comfortable and enjoyable external conditions. If we want to find the perfect partner, a new job, a nice home, attract wealth then all we have to do is set our intention and "the universe" will send these things to us. This sounds too good to be true but Reiki can actually work for us in this way for a time and consequently this is how many people use this precious and sacred energy.

Reiki can give us great power to achieve our personal goals there is no doubt about this. However, power without wisdom can be dangerous and will not last. Everyone experiences this phenomenon to a different extent. For some people Reiki will work in this way for a whole lifetime, for others maybe a few years, for some maybe only a few months, intermittently, or not at all. Why is this so and what is the downside of using Reiki in a controlling or materialistic way?

Like all things in life it comes back to the universal laws of karma. Many people now have the karma to encounter and experience Reiki because of our good actions in previous lives. Our experience of the power and potential of Reiki is directly linked to our actions in previous lives. The extent to which we can receive or benefit from Reiki in this life also accords with the quality and quantity of these past positive or negative mental (thoughts and feelings), verbal (speech), and physical actions and the intention/motivation behind them.

On the face of it we might think that someone who is easily able to use Reiki to attract beautiful partners, a high income, a stable family life, and so on is very fortunate and must have been very kind and virtuous in previous lives. The latter no doubt is true but the former is very doubtful. When we have used up all our karma for good external conditions in this life only difficulties await us. We can actually use Reiki in this way to use up all our good karma more quickly and this can create a dangerous situation for us.

This may be a difficult concept to accept but a human life or rebirth is very rare and difficult to obtain. If we use up all our karma for being human our next rebirth will not be as a human being. So if we spend our life "feathering our own nest" and use this special and sacred energy to help us do this, all we are really doing is accelerating our own demise.

Those people who are not too bothered about obtaining comfortable external conditions and find it easy to develop pure inner realizations and pure spiritual teachers are really the most fortunate beings. These people who have an interest in the spiritual path and a sincere wish to help others are creating unimaginable good conditions for themselves in the future. Although they are using up good karma all the time that they are in human form, as we all are, this is more than offset by the good karma that they are creating for the future. So we have to be really careful how we use our time on Earth. In the great scheme of things a human life is really quite short but if we use it wisely and compassionately we can set ourselves up for an eternity of inner peace, universal wisdom, bliss, and wonder, and the opportunity to guide others toward the same state.

This really is a major Reiki lesson to learn. If all Reiki teachers had the courage to share this with their students we could avoid many problems in the future. As it is nowadays there are many Reiki people inadvertently enjoying temporary good fortune whilst storing up many problems for themselves in the future.

Wisdom is the answer to all our problems, understanding the way things are, the way things work – how our minds work, how the "laws of the universe" work, how we should live our lives if we want to find lasting happiness for ourselves and others. How wonderful it would be if we lived in a world where learning these truths were simply a natural part of growing up. How wonderful it would be if everyone had access to this knowledge and could live their lives accordingly and experience great happiness because of it. A pipedream? Maybe, maybe not, that depends upon your mind and you can change that whenever you like!

We can summarize the laws of cause and effect or karma in four lines:

- All our good actions of body, speech, and mind create good karma for the future.
- All our negative/selfish actions create unpleasant karma for the future.
- All the pleasurable things we experience use up good karma.
- All the unpleasant things we experience (especially if we can maintain peaceful/patient mind) use up bad karma, then we will never have to experience that particular problem again.

So we can see that all our negative actions will result in unpleasant experiences and all our good actions will result in pleasant experiences. However, there are further implications such as the fact that all our actions create mental tendencies or habits in the mind. So good intentions and actions will create the tendency for us to do similar actions in the future.

The karma we create now will also dictate the type of body and realm/world and the type of environment we will be born into in future lives. We might take a higher or lower rebirth, maybe with a healthy body and mind if we are fortunate, and the environment might be pleasant and peaceful or violent and deadly, depending on what type of karma ripens when we die. The law of karma is a fascinating and in-depth subject; if you want an authentic, detailed but very accessible explanation try one of the books listed in Appendix 5.

We might think that future lives are a long way off and that they will take care of themselves so we can just enjoy ourselves now and not worry about such things. But the reality is that our next life might only be a breath away, we do not know for sure. Generally we feel as if we will live forever and we rarely consider our own mortality. But it is vital that we do think about death every day if we want to make the most of our life. Considering and realizing that our grip on life is very tenuous forces us to make the most of each day, to really appreciate life, to try to create good karma every day and, most importantly, to look for some kind of refuge or antidote to death, and what might come after, before it is too late. One simple antidote is learning to develop and hold a peaceful and compassionate mind. If we can cultivate such a mind throughout our life and maintain it whilst we are dying, sincerely wishing to use our future lives to follow a pure spiritual path and help others as much as possible, then this will definitely help us find the right kind of rebirth to fulfill these wishes. Whenever others are dying we can help them by encouraging them to keep a peaceful mind, to pray, to think of the welfare of others, to stay relaxed and positive. All these types of mind at the time of death encourage good karma to ripen and will help them to take a fortunate rebirth. Of course we do not want to overdo it at such times and often just having someone in the room who is relaxed and positive is all that they need to feel the same, especially if we are quietly giving them Reiki as well. When someone is close to the moment of death we can gently stroke or touch the crown of their head and this will encourage the subtle mind to leave the body through this part off the body. This also helps to ensure a fortunate rebirth.

Why are the laws of karma relevant to Reiki? Well at the heart of Dr. Usui's teaching practice were the Five Principles and also we now know that he used traditional Japanese Waka poetry to teach his students how to live their lives with Reiki. The poetry and principles are basically spiritual guidelines emphasizing the importance of leading a good life, trying to develop some wisdom and compassion, and not using Reiki with a selfish or harmful attitude. Basically, how to live a meaningful life, one that aspires to goodness, virtue, and honesty. We can all aspire to these qualities. We have to work on ourselves a little every day; if some days we do not make much progress, no problem, don't worry. Simply to aspire, to try, is creating great karma for the future; in time we will find it much easier to develop and attain pure spiritual realizations. But if we don't try we won't make any headway and in future lives we will find it even harder to make the effort.

The original Reiki principles

Looking back, the main purpose of Reiho was not only to heal diseases, but also to have right mind and healthy body so that people would enjoy and experience happiness in life. Therefore when it comes to teaching, first let the student understand well the Meiji Emperor's admonitory, then in the morning and in the evening let them chant and have in mind the five precepts which are:

First we say, today don't get angry.
Secondly we say, don't worry.
Third we say, be thankful.
Fourth we say, endeavor your work.
Fifth we say, be kind to people.

(My friend Emiko Arai was very firm about the above wording.)
This is truly a very important admonitory. This is the same way wisemen and saints disciplined themselves since ancient times. Sensei named these the "secret methods of inviting happiness", "the spiritual medicine of many diseases" to clarify his purpose to teach. Moreover, his intention was that a teaching method should be as simple as possible and not difficult to understand. Every morning and every evening, sit still in silence with your hands in prayer (gassho) and chant the affirmations, then a pure and healthy mind would be nurtured. It was the true meaning of this to practice this in daily life, using it. (i.e. put it into practical use) This is the reason why Reiho became so popular. (see the Usui Precepts for more on this.)

Extract from Dr. Usui's memorial inscription

The fact that Mikao Usui requires that his students repeat and contemplate these principles twice a day is also an indication that they are a very important part of the practice. If we can work out a way to incorporate them into our daily practice they are another way of deepening our relationship with Reiki. We can recite them silently before a treatment if we wish and also visualize Dr. Usui or another being like Jesus or Buddha. We can also imagine that he (or our own spiritual guide) is with us while we are giving treatments, a very special way of strengthening our connection with him and Reiki.

If we set a little time aside each morning and evening to recite these principles, give ourselves a little Reiki, pray and/or meditate a little this will greatly improve our experience of Reiki. We will find we generally have more energy and peace of mind and our life has more harmony or synchronicity to it. This is a sign that we are living in accordance with Reiki, that we are actually allowing this wonderful energy to enter our lives and color all our experiences with its infinite peace and beauty.

Also the fact that Mikao Usui encouraged his students to actively seek and develop their own inner potential indicates that such practices practically support and enhance our use of Reiki as a healing technique.

If we don't practice a daily meditation or pray or recite the Reiki principles will our experience of Reiki become weaker? This depends upon the frequency and the way we use Reiki, our motivation, our state of mind, and our karma. If we are regularly using Reiki in a very positive way to help others and we have a sincere wish to improve our good qualities then our experience of Reiki can only improve.

Occasionally we might feel a little "flat." Perhaps we sometimes don't feel the powerful presence of Reiki when we want it, but this is simply part of the path. Often at these times Reiki is saying now it is your turn to make an effort! When we work through these times we often emerge stronger, clearer, and more complete beings. Sometimes we can really benefit from difficult circumstances if we use them to develop good qualities like patience, empathy, kindness, etc. If the path were always smooth and downhill we would soon become weak and dependent on others stronger than ourselves and that is not a healthy way to live. We can also become of great benefit to others through experiencing and walking this path before them. A new path through a dense forest is always difficult to make, but the more people that walk that way the clearer the path becomes, and the easier it becomes for others who follow.

If our mind degenerates our experience of Reiki will degenerate. If we become more selfish and proud, more concerned for our own welfare, our relationship with Reiki will weaken because we are pulling away from Reiki. If we are doing the opposite and genuinely trying to develop our good qualities, the same qualities that Reiki possesses, we are actively moving toward Reiki and so the quality of the energy we "carry" will only become purer.

We cannot imagine what level of energy or state of mind such beings as Jesus or Buddha reflect, their nature is the very perfection of all good qualities. All their teachings emphasized the development of wisdom, compassion, faith, devotion to the welfare of others, etc. So it is obvious that if we wish to heal as they did we need to become like them in personality. This seems like an impossibly tall order, but it is definitely possible, as they said many times themselves. All the great spiritual teachers, all the fully enlightened beings, were at one time just like us, lost and confused, trying to make sense of everything. The only difference was they made a firm decision and applied strong and consistent effort to grasp the essence of their life, to begin and complete the spiritual path. We now have a special opportunity to do as they have done.

If we really want to do this we need to find a spiritual path that we are sure will lead us to full enlightenment and we need to find a teacher or spiritual guide who can show us how to begin, steadily progress, and complete this path either in this life or as soon as possible. If we don't look for and find these two things we will not be able to become fully enlightened. Unfortunately enlightenment will not naturally arise in our minds, we cannot accidentally stumble across it, and we cannot develop it without knowing the correct methods. Even if we lead a good life and go out of our way to create great amounts of good karma, at some point in our future lives this karma will run out and we are back where we started or worse.

Finally it is worth mentioning that our daily practice of reciting the five principles, if we choose to pursue this, should not become a chore, as then it will lose its special power to improve our Reiki practice. So if we cannot change our mind we need to be flexible and on some days vary the practice a little. Just concentrate on one principle perhaps, or just pray, just give yourself some Reiki, read a spiritual text, and so on. It is also worth mentioning that if we use too many different techniques we can lose our way a little. Sometimes it is better to work through our boredom or discouragement and try to break through this barrier to a new level of understanding.

Also the spiritual path is a middle way, we should not be lazy and expect Reiki to do all the work but we should not become an aesthetic with a hard militaristic outlook. Being hard on ourselves is just another way of sabotaging our spiritual progression. We need to make a daily effort to improve ourselves but try to keep a light, happy, content, and flexible mind. When we need to rest, rest, and when we need to motivate ourselves, motivate. When difficulties arise in our life or in our spiritual practice just try to accept them with a light and peaceful mind; they will pass much more quickly. Actually accepting problems with a sincerely peaceful and happy mind is in itself a profound spiritual practice, a special way of training the mind and the most powerful way of purifying negative karma that has already arisen in our lives. However, this is not an excuse to put on a brave face as this generally is not very wise or helpful! Always a middle way.

3

Two of the most frequently asked questions by first degree Reiki students are "do I need to take second degree?" and "how is it different from first degree?" The answer to the first question is obviously "no." First degree Reiki is an excellent healing system, complete in itself. Quite simply the more we use our first degree skills the more we will develop our healing abilities for our own and others' benefit. We can carry on like this for the rest of our life if we feel that we are happy with this level of practice and rate of spiritual progression.

Spiritual progression

Another point to bear in mind is that we all come to Reiki at a different point in our spiritual progression so, and this might seem a little strange, Reiki Masters of considerable experience might find themselves teaching first degree students who are far more spiritually advanced than themselves! This is not always obvious, however, as advanced spiritual qualities are quite subtle and we have to have a very clear mind to recognize them. Advanced spiritual qualities are not things like being able to predict the future or read others' minds, many people have these abilities but are generally no more happy or content than others. Such abilities can be a great obstacle to real spiritual progression as they can promote pride and a sense of self-importance or superiority over others. Pure spiritual qualities are really simple and quite subtle to our normally gross view of the world. Just things like being humble, patient, concern for others' welfare, honesty, good manners, courage, and wisdom are the qualities that will lead to us to higher spiritual realizations because these qualities are in themselves close to the qualities of an enlightened being. Actually if we work to develop these qualities we will find that such things as clairvoyance and healing abilities eventually come quite naturally. Then, because of our good inner qualities, we will know how and when to use these gifts to really benefit others. Using such gifts without wisdom can actually stunt our spiritual growth and when other people see this they can lose faith in the spiritual path because of our poor example. On Dr. Usui's memorial stone it actually says "he was a warm, simple, and humble person" so we can see this as an excellent example of what we can achieve in our lives if we simply concentrate on developing our good qualities and trying to lessen our tendencies toward selfishness.

It is worth passing on this advice at this point because some second degree practitioners experience an increase in their psychic abilities and if we want to develop these abilities further the best way to do this is, rather than doing many complicated mental exercises, is simply, as mentioned, to be more kind, loving, giving, etc. Deep heartfelt compassion really purifies the mind; advanced spiritual practitioners can verify this. The purer the mind the clearer all our senses and awarenesses become. Ultimately we can purify the mind to such a degree that we become blissfully awakened or enlightened. We become omniscient, seeing all things clearly and simultaneously and we become completely focused on helping others find lasting happiness. But trying to develop psychic abilities for our own benefit will only take us away from this. Actually we can only attain enlightenment if our motivation is to benefit others.

Most of the things we do with a selfish motivation will eventually lead us to experience suffering. Conversely anything we do for others' benefit will lead to good fortune and can be a cause of our own enlightenment, especially if this is our intention. Coming back to the question of how second degree differs from first degree, this is not so easy to answer as, apart from the obvious differences such as the use of symbols, the main difference is the experience of the second degree "energy." This is a very personal thing and if you ask ten second degree practitioners they may all describe it differently. Common experiences are that the energy feels finer or more subtle or that it seems to work on a deeper level than first degree. Also issues seem to be resolved faster and more smoothly, physical and mental healing can also be accelerated, and there is a general sense that the practitioner is closer to the "source" of Reiki.

Practitioners also experience clearer self-understanding and gain clarity on other personal issues like relationships and their own path in life. Generally all the benefits that we experience with first degree are accelerated and amplified, very broadly we can say that the energy is about four times more powerful than first degree. The degree to which we find this to be true differs with the individual, some people are deeply touched by the second degree attunements and subsequent practice. They can change greatly within themselves and decide to make many changes in their lives. For many though the changes are more subtle, although still very powerful. Because it is quite difficult to see our own mind it is often others who bring such inner changes to our attention or we may find ourselves only recognizing amazing inner changes when we look back over the first few months since taking second degree.

The story of second degree Reiki

Before we became more aware of the Japanese Reiki tradition it was widely believed in the West that Dr. Usui received the symbols at the end of a 21-day retreat. According to the story, during a special spiritual experience, induced through extensive meditation, the symbols appeared to him in "bubbles" of light and their meaning and how to use them was also "transmitted." We cannot be sure if this is what actually happened, as this story is not verified in the Japanese tradition. However, we know that he was a practicing Buddhist and that meditation retreats would have been a regular part of his spiritual practice and we know from Dr. Usui's memorial inscription that "One day he [Dr. Usui] went to Mount Kurama on a 21-day retreat to fast and meditate. At the end of this period he suddenly felt the great Reiki energy at the top of his head, which led to the Reiki healing system."

There is no mention of him having been given symbols during this mystical experience and the general feeling now is that he introduced the symbols, structured teaching system, and methods for attunements later on in order to share Reiki with others and help people to use it as effectively as possible. Perhaps he was guided or inspired by Reiki to do this. This is borne out by the fact that some Reiki symbols are very similar to those used in Buddhism, Shintoism and some simply relate to Japanese Kanji or writing. Nevertheless they are now sacred symbols in the Reiki tradition and should be regarded as such in order to preserve and prolong the purity of this tradition. It is really wonderful to know that the Reiki Dr. Usui first experienced on Mount Kurama and tried on himself, family, and friends, before teaching it further afield, is the same Reiki we receive and can share with others.

Meditation on original Reiki

If we want to create a special link with Dr. Usui and the first time he received Reiki, sit in a chair and put your hands on your body, either over your heart or somewhere comfortable like your thighs. After a few minutes of quiet imagine your crown chakra opens like a lotus flower, visualize a small six-inch-size Dr. Usui hovering over your crown in meditation posture and smiling, also emitting infinite rays of white and golden light/Reiki. Imagine your body and mind fill with this light and mentally repeat "Reiki" three times. Try to feel the wise and loving presence of Dr. Usui and ask him to bless your mind. Imagine what it was like when Dr. Usui first received Reiki on Mount Kurama, imagine that you are there and receiving Reiki for the first time as he did. Then make a simple commitment to use Reiki wisely, to help others, and develop your own good qualities in order to benefit others as Dr. Usui did. A good intention is simply something like "healthy mind, healthy body, meaningful life." Again, we can quietly say this three times. When you have finished imagine the blessings you have received are sealed within your mind. If you have a special place like a local hilltop, a favorite tree, a wood, or near a river or stream this can be a lovely place to do this meditation.

Whenever we do some kind of spiritual practice like this or whenever we do something to help others, however small, we can dedicate or direct the positive energy or good karma created by our actions for the benefit of others. This stops the power of our good karma degenerating and actually increases it so that the karmic benefits that return to us in the future are greater. We can simply think "through the power of my positive actions may all beings find lasting happiness" or "through the good potential of this virtuous action may all beings attain the happiness of full enlightenment swiftly and easily."

Dr. Usui may have introduced the different degrees or levels of practice in order to help people progress gradually and consistently and to give people something to aim for or wish to attain. This would have helped their spiritual practice become smooth and enjoyable. Also Dr. Usui must have been meditating for years before he attained Reiki so we can assume that the different levels of Reiki probably lead up to what he experienced on Mount Kurama. If we tried to go straight to that level of awareness our minds probably couldn't cope with the experience. Once an enlightened teacher said that he could take a man to full enlightenment in six days, the people who were listening to him were amazed. Then he said the only problem is that it would then take ten men to hold him down! So it is right that we progress gradually and comfortably toward our goal, if we are on the right path there is no rush, and if we practice within our capacity and with consistent effort the outcome is assured.

The value of second degree Reiki

It is very difficult to give Reiki a monetary value. Nowadays Masters charge different rates and some charge nothing at all. There are valid arguments for both ways of presenting Reiki and these have been discussed at length in many books. It is interesting that in the Tibetan Buddhist tradition spiritual practitioners pay very little for being able to receive the most profound and powerful empowerments. They are available for anyone who has a sincere wish to practice that particular type of meditation or for those who wish to simply receive the profound blessings of a particular Buddha whom they feel a close connection with. However, because these empowerments are given within the context of a spiritual framework, which constantly teaches how special and rare they are, there is less danger of taking them for granted. Buddhists generally know that a human life is not easily obtained and that a human life with the opportunity to follow a pure spiritual path to enlightenment is incredibly rare. They also understand that we create great negative karma if we disrespect pure holy teachings and teachers.

However, with Reiki, because the techniques are passed on to the student in a short space of time we don't have much time to contemplate or deeply understand the value of what we are receiving. So because we in the West have a strong understanding of the value of money, paying an appropriate fee can help us think about the value of Reiki. This is even more important in Western Reiki as in Japan the process of teaching first degree was and still is combined with in-depth spiritual teaching, which helps the student understand the value of Reiki, which in turn deepens faith and improves results. If the Master was not satisfied that the student was ready to receive Reiki the attunements would be postponed until the student was ready.

In fact most Japanese Reiki practitioners are simply first degree practitioners. Not many people progress to second degree and even fewer go higher, simply because of the level of commitment required. Whereas in the West anyone can become a Reiki Master in a matter of weeks! Maybe Western Reiki has developed in this way for a reason. We cannot say for sure that Western Reiki is inferior because of these facts; things have just evolved differently in the West. Eventually traditional Japanese Reiki practitioners will be commonplace in the West and then we can choose what feels right for us. There are no rules, if we feel ready to move on to a new level of Reiki training within a few months of the last level of training we can do this. If we want to learn slowly and traditionally this is fine also. Reiki is Reiki whatever form it takes; we simply have to find what feels right for us.

Whether we learn quickly or slowly really appreciating or trying to grasp the real value of second degree will greatly help our practice. So it is best to think deeply about whether we are ready to take second degree. Deep appreciation of Reiki will change our attitude toward it, which will change our experience.

Why use symbols?

It is well known that the two main purposes of second degree Reiki, are to enable the practitioner to improve healing on a mental and emotional level and to facilitate absentee or long-distance healing. Both of these can be done with first degree but to a much more accomplished level in second degree. There are many other things we can do with the techniques we learn in second degree and these all involve the use of sacred symbols.

Some symbols are very simple and easily recognizable. They can have a very powerful meaning and can invoke strong mental and emotional reactions. For example, a cross is a very simple symbol, consisting of only two straight lines, but the meaning and connotations of such a symbol can be enormous, depending of course on the mind that perceives it. If you had never seen a cross before it would have no meaning to you, but if you are a Christian it can have a profound and deeply spiritual meaning. So as with most things the power of any symbol depends upon the mind that perceives it. All the "qualities" that external objects appear to possess are merely imputed or projected by our mind or consciousness. But generally this happens without us being consciously aware of it! We see a person, an object, an environment and at the very same moment we subconsciously project certain qualities, good, bad, or indifferent on to such things and then we believe that these qualities are truly part of the object or person. In fact we are very mistaken in our view of reality and we will look at this more closely later on as an understanding of the true nature of reality is crucial if we are serious about the spiritual path to real freedom and lasting happiness.

We will look later at the meaning and beauty of symbols but for now it is interesting to note that Reiki symbols do have a special meaning to Reiki practitioners as they are used in and form a special part of the attunement process. So when we see them for the first time we already have a close relationship with them. They are almost already part of us.

Authentic Reiki

It is now well known that Reiki Masters use symbols as part of the attunement process. In fact the symbols themselves and the actual process of attunements have been published in books and on the Internet. This has been widely condemned, but maybe no real harm has been done. It has not affected the power and effectiveness of Reiki; at worst perhaps it has taken away a little of the mystery and magic for those coming to Reiki for the first time. We need to be patient, kind, and tolerant toward others always, and if a few Reiki teachers are not playing the game we have to accept this. A negative attitude toward others is never a solution. If anything it should help us to keep our own commitments to original Reiki more strongly.

Possession of the symbols and the knowledge of the attunement process cannot create a Reiki Master or an advanced or second degree practitioner. We need to receive the attunements from a Master who has a clear unbroken lineage to Dr. Usui. Almost all Reiki Masters do have this clear link so we can be sure that what we are receiving is genuine and authentic Reiki. Without the attunements the symbols have little or no power as Reiki symbols. The only power they would possess in such a case is the power we mentally project on to them or believe that they have. However, once we receive the symbols as part of a Reiki attunement they become embedded in our subconscious mind and when we see them or use them the healing we can receive and give works on and from this very deep subtle level.

The Japanese equivalent of second degree Reiki is called Okuden, which translates as "deeper knowledge." This is an indication that second degree and the higher levels of Reiki are not just tools for healing but really the beginnings of a very special path to healing on all levels of body, mind, and spirit. It is really primarily a spiritual path although many of us might have resistance to such a suggestion and prefer to describe it as a path to personal growth or something similar. Either way if we embark on such a journey and take the essence of second degree Reiki to heart all the benefits we received from first degree will be greatly enhanced. We will find that we become even more in tune with Reiki. We will experience deeper levels of contentment in our lives and our relationships will become more harmonious, especially if we are giving or sending Reiki to others.

If we have a faith or religion it will be greatly enriched with second degree, our faith may become deeper and we may feel closer to God or to our own higher nature or however we define the "greatest good." Consequently second degree may help us to change direction in life, giving more clarity to our own mission or purpose in life, whatever that may be. Gradually, with consistent practice, we shall become more able to see ourselves, how our mind works, our good and bad habits. And most importantly second degree empowers us to take control of ourselves, to gradually reduce our negative patterns and enhance our good qualities. We can see ourselves in a new light.

To some extent this will happen quite naturally as our practice progresses, but we can take a much more active role in this process of self-discovery simply by regularly setting our intent to "see the truth in all things" to "see ourselves as we really are" and to "realize our full potential for the greatest good." When we know where we are and where we want to go we can move toward that goal. But if we never look "within" our life will always be shallow and our achievements will be superficial. It is very easy nowadays to spend our whole life being busy, achieving many external goals. These goals may even appear to be altruistic like healing others, teaching, and other public services but we can easily overlook the real meaning of life if we are forever busy. A human life is so rare and quite brief in the great scheme of things so we have to be really careful how we use our time. If we were told we only had a few months to live we would suddenly stop and think very carefully how best to use the time we had left. This is how we should approach the rest of our life because firstly we really do not know how much time we have left and even if we do reach a good age the time will pass very quickly. So we need to check carefully that what we are doing with our life has some real meaning and value then we can look forward to a really bright future in this life and those to come.

Although many second degree practitioners report amazing changes in themselves and their lives during or soon after the attunements what we really want to be trying to achieve is long-term, consistent, and steady progress. Amazing spiritual experiences can be very exciting but sooner or later we have to deal with the realities of daily life. Developing simple good qualities, as taught by Jesus, Buddha, Krisha, Mohammed, etc., is the essence of the path to full enlightenment or simply the path to lasting happiness. Again if we gently work on our own mind in this way using Reiki to help us and try to help others do the same then we are really doing something special with our lives. Also amazing spiritual experiences will come to us quite naturally as a byproduct of our good inner work. But if we purposefully seek spiritual highs for our own amusement, although temporarily fulfilling, this will just bring us many problems in the future and can just be another addiction or distraction.

Simple good qualities like trying to live joyfully, lovingly, honestly, courageously, kindly, compassionately, wisely, patiently, humbly are the real stepping-stones across the river of life's problems. If we don't treasure and try to develop these qualities we may simply be swept away.

The cycle of suffering

Buddha taught that all living beings go from one life to another again and again, endlessly experiencing the difficulties of birth, ageing, sickness, and death, being parted from those we love, not being able to fulfill our wishes, having to endure all kinds of mental and physical problems. Sometimes we are reborn as animals, ghosts, gods, humans, and other kinds of beings. There are countless different types of rebirth, most of which are characterized by sufferings of one sort or another. Even those lives that are pleasant eventually end in sickness and death and probably then we have to face the misfortune of an unpleasant rebirth. This cycle of suffering is a manifestation of our karma from previous lives. We cannot find a start to this cycle, although we do not remember we have been in it since beginningless time. Unless we acknowledge these truths and make an effort to escape we will have countless future lives all in the nature of suffering and confusion, depicted on page 33.

This is a huge concept for us to grasp and it is easy to dismiss it as part of an ancient religious belief. But if we think about it carefully and read good explanations (see Appendix 5) we may come to feel and know that this is the truth and that we and those we love are in a precarious situation and that now is the time to do something about it!

Buddhists believe that a human life is like a holiday from the cycle of suffering; we cannot remember the fear and hunger of being a wild animal or the mental torture of being a lost ghost so we live our lives as though there is no danger of returning to such a state of existence. But there is real danger of this every moment of our life. So this is why the spiritual path is so important, and why it is really the most important aspect of Reiki. Buddha said that a human life, especially one where we have an interest in the spiritual path, is like a boat that enables us to cross the river of suffering. If we want to escape from the cycle of life, death, and rebirth and attain enlightenment we need to develop a strong and consistent wish to escape by recognizing these dangers for ourselves. Then with this powerful motivation we try to develop and perfect our good qualities like compassion and wisdom, which is the essence of all pure spiritual traditions – the actual path to enlightenment. Only enlightened beings have the wisdom and power to fully protect others from suffering so ultimately if we want to be of real benefit to others this should be our goal.

It is important though not to feel that we have to take on this view if we are not comfortable with it. We can just put such things to one side and just take from this book what is of practical benefit to us at present.

From the point of view of Reiki if we are trying to develop our good qualities and help others do the same we are going in the right direction. All religions and genuine spiritual paths will point us in the right direction if we practice, patiently, consistently, happily and with the wish to help others. Then when our own death comes we will be happy and relaxed and feeling content with a life well spent.

Many people feel Buddhism in its purest form is simply truism, it

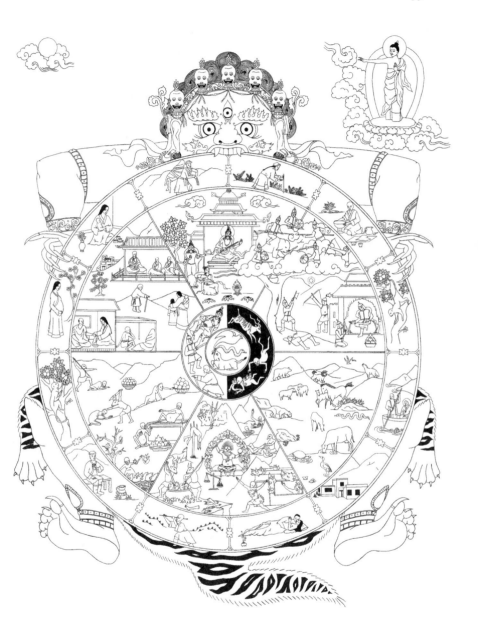

The 'wheel of life'

tells us the way things are, why we are here, how we got here, what to expect in the future, how we can solve our daily problems, and how to avoid any kind of suffering in the future. If you want to know more about Buddhism see Appendix 4.

Conscious Reiki

One of the most exciting and empowering aspects of second degree Reiki is that we are able to take a much more active role in the healing process and in our own process of personal growth or gradual enlightenment. We are given the tools and techniques to accelerate our learning and experiencing of the inner path to self-knowledge and lasting happiness and we can use these special gifts to help others in many ways.

Symbols are used in many religions and spiritual traditions for different purposes and the language and use of symbols is explained in the next chapter. This is a very interesting and profound subject but not difficult to understand and use to great effect in our everyday life.

One of the main qualities of the higher levels of Reiki training is that we learn how to work with the energy rather than just being a channel for the energy. The conscious intentions that we use to do this bring us closer to the essence of Reiki. We become much more aware of how Reiki is working with and through us to improve our own life and those around us and this is a wonderful experience.

As with first degree Reiki the more practice we have of using the higher levels the more we will learn and the faster we will progress. If we learn second degree but decide not to use the symbols or we feel they do not conform to our religious beliefs we will still gain great benefit from receiving the attunements and carrying the higher energy. However, we should not be put off from using the symbols because these teachings seem too esoteric or weird! The symbols are really an outward manifestation of Reiki. They are simply keys to higher Reiki and we probably know from our own experience of Reiki that it is "all good" so we need not worry that we are dabbling with something strange.

Reiki at the speed of light!

Second degree Reiki practitioners can give themselves a full treatment in half the time it takes first degree practitioners. We use the same twelve hand positions but instead of five minutes in each position we spend two and a half minutes or just two if we are pushed for time. Of course we can still treat ourselves for a full hour if we wish and when we are treating others, especially if they are not second degree practitioners, a full hour is often preferable. One of the obvious advantages of being able to work more quickly and on a deeper level is that if we only have ten or fifteen minutes to give someone Reiki the power of that treatment can be greatly increased. Also when we learn how to use the symbols we can achieve remarkable levels of healing in only a short time and we can use the symbols to ensure that the patient continues to receive Reiki long after we have physically left their presence.

We will also find that the absentee or long-distance techniques for sending Reiki are very powerful. The use of symbols can make an absentee treatment at least as powerful as being physically present with the patient. When we experience sending and receiving long-distance Reiki for the first time it is amazing to feel the strength and presence of the energy. It seems to just appear out of thin air! Many Reiki and non-Reiki people become aware of this when someone is sending them Reiki without a prearranged time. We can be walking down the street minding our own business when we feel the energy switch on as someone has just decided to send us a full treatment! Reiki is incredibly flexible in this way and with a little imagination we can use our new-found skills to do wonderful things for others and have great fun trying this out and playing with the energy.

The purpose of higher degree

Why did Dr. Usui teach higher levels of Reiki? Simply for the same reason as he shared first degree Reiki with others: because he wanted others to be happy and healthy, and to find some lasting peace of mind and contentment. This is what he himself experienced with Reiki so it was natural to want others to enjoy this as well. He did not teach Reiki to become a rich man or for fame or fortune. He did not seek the acclaim of others, he simply wanted to share his happiness with others.

Dr. Usui wrote down the Five Reiki Principles and gave each of his students a copy to take home. The title of the original page, written in his own handwriting, reads,

The secret method for inviting happiness

and then the subtitle reads

the wonderful method for all diseases (of body and mind)

The essence of Reiki and especially the higher levels of Reiki is very simple. It is really just about finding happiness, lasting happiness from within. What do we generally experience when we give and receive Reiki? Definitely some inner peace and freedom from our daily problems. Our levels of stress lessen and we become more content, alert, clear minded, patient, loving, we smile more easily. If we have ever been to a Reiki exchange then we know this is generally how we feel afterwards. We leave showing all the symptoms of a happy mind!

All living beings are looking for happiness. This is the main motivation behind all our actions. We are constantly, consciously and subconsciously, seeking happiness and trying to avoid problems. This motivation is such a natural part of our makeup that we generally do not notice it. But if we think deeply about it we will realize that all our decisions in life are controlled by the wish to find happiness and avoid problems. What career we choose, our partner, our car, our house, even just small decisions like which brand of jam or what kind of bread to buy are motivated by our constant wish to obtain what we like and avoid what we do not like. Even suicide is motivated by the wish to find peace of mind and avoid the pain of life.

If we try to swat a fly what does it do? It flies away, it has no wish to be harmed and wishes to live and fulfill its desires. Humans and animals and all living beings live like this and yet it is very rare in this world for someone to find lasting happiness. We all look for happiness in the external world. We rely on many people and things to bring us happiness. We do not realize how much this is true. Try to imagine being separated from the things you rely on like friends and family, money, possessions, good health, etc., and try to imagine the amount of pain and stress you would experience if some of these things were taken away from you. This indicates how much we rely on these things to be happy.

If we look around at the people we work or live with, the people in our neighborhood, or the people we pass on the street it is hard to find someone who is truly, deeply, and consistently happy. Happiness is simply an inner quality, a state of mind that arises from within and yet we constantly look for it externally. If we wish to find lasting happiness we must begin by acknowledging this simple but very powerful truth.

When through receiving or giving Reiki we feel happy and relaxed what has happened, why do we feel content and peaceful? Quite simply our mind has changed. Without relying on an external phenomenon like another person, new car, new clothes, etc. we have found some happiness from within. If we could "access" this happiness on a daily basis and familiarize ourselves with it and where it comes from then our general level of happiness, contentment, and quality of life will continually increase. Understanding and experiencing this timeless truth is ultimately the answer to all our problems and forms the basis of the path to liberation from suffering.

The essence of Reiki and especially the higher levels is about

finding happiness from a different source and going out of our
way to share this with others whenever possible. If we regard Reiki
simply as a healing technique that is what it will be for us. If we wish
to look a little deeper into the true nature of things, face the facts
of life, and look for some lasting solution to our own and others'
daily problems then, applied with a little wisdom, Reiki can take us
a long way toward our ultimate potential.

A branch of the Buddha tree

It is very helpful to keep these truths in mind while learning
about and practicing the higher levels of Reiki. A good motivation
is really helpful. If we use Reiki with the intention of finding
happiness in the external world by attracting the perfect partner,
the best job, more money, etc., we might find some short-term
increase in the quality of our external life. Ultimately though,
selfish thoughts and intentions create the causes for problems
and unhappiness in the future. As mentioned earlier we can use
Reiki to manifest good external conditions but this uses up vast
amounts of good karma and if our motivation is selfish it creates
much negative karma.

If we use Reiki to help us train our mind and develop our good
qualities this will help us find some inner peace and happiness in
the short term and it will create much positive karma resulting in
many good things coming our way in future lives. Also if we develop
the virtuous intention of training our mind with the wish to help
others do the same then this creates unimaginable good karma for
ourselves and for others. Another way of changing our motivation
with regard to our daily use of Reiki is to simply regularly think
"this Reiki I carry, I carry for others" or "may all my Reiki actions
be a cause for the happiness and welfare of others" or anything
similar. The more we familiarize our mind with doing things with
the motivation to benefit others the more powerful our actions will
become and the deeper and more genuine our compassion will

become. Developing our compassion and wisdom is the essence of the path to enlightenment. Ultimately the only way we can solve all our problems is by attaining enlightenment and yet we can only attain enlightenment by abandoning selfish wishes/intentions and developing and perfecting our wish to help others!

So we can see that we have to be wise with our use of Reiki. Dr. Usui would have had great understanding of the laws of karma and the value of using Reiki for the right reasons and in ways that will bring lasting inner benefits. We might have lost a little of this understanding in the West, but things are changing and we are developing a more complete picture of how to use Reiki in the wisest and most beneficial ways.

At the end of Dr. Usui's written script presenting the Five Principles to his students he concludes by saying that Reiki is "for the improvement of body and soul," not for the accumulation of wealth and reputation!

4

Transforming addictive behavior

One of the special qualities of second degree Reiki is the enhanced ability it gives us for mental and emotional healing. With this in mind one of the most common ways in which we will use our new-found skills is in helping ourselves and others to break negative thought patterns and addictive behavior. This might take the form of depression, grief, persistent anger, loneliness, lack of confidence, or simply any unhappy emotion or repetitive thoughts that we cannot prevent disturbing our peace of mind.

Since the mind is a creature of habit we can see that people who are consistently happy and content with their lot in life have developed a kind of positive addiction to this enjoyable mental and emotional experience. Whereas those who generally have a bleak view of life or who are consistently impatient, irritable, or generally moody have got so used to being this way that it is quite difficult for them to change and act differently. This is a classic sign of addictive behavior. Basically the further down the line or the more we allow these habits to continue the more difficult it will be to change. We have to make an effort to change and create familiarity with positivity and contentment now in order to reap the rewards of natural happiness in the future. People who naturally have a happy and peaceful mind are experiencing the good karma of having made an effort to improve their mind in previous lives. As explained later we can change our minds, we do not have to accept ourselves as we are especially if that is causing us to be unhappy.

Obviously there are more gross or obvious types of addictive behavior like drinking, taking drugs, being attracted to abusive relationships, etc, and with second degree comes the ability to offer people a real opportunity to transform their mind and therefore their life. The second degree symbols are the "keys" to this wonderful healing work and learning to use them and beginning to understand how they work is a fascinating journey.

Beyond time and space

Second degree Reiki is a very powerful personal transformational technique. It is powerful enough for us to be able to manipulate our environment and manifest those things that we wish to attract or manifest. So as previously discussed we have a responsibility to acquire a little wisdom through our own experience and through reading and talking with our Reiki friends and teachers. When we develop this wisdom we will come to understand that the most effective and wisest way to use Reiki is simply as an aid to personal growth and spiritual development, to help others develop in the same way and of course as a healing technique for body and mind. Although this might seem like three different purposes in practice they are interdependent facets of Reiki. Reiki simply works to increase our inner happiness and the outer benefits are an added bonus.

When we feel we are ready to move up a gear and take second degree we will discover a whole new world of Reiki. From simply using Reiki as a "hands on" technique we are thrown in to a world of clearer, higher, more subtle energy levels, a world of self-revelation and advances in personal growth. This new world can shake our conceptions of time and space as the symbols unlock the mind and give us great power to accelerate our spiritual development and healing potential.

The nature of reality

At the moment we live in a "solid" world, things appear very "real" to us. Our body, our environment, our relationships and possessions all seem very real! It seems that we are often powerless to change things for the better, that we and others are trapped within this apparently solid reality. We may also feel that our character or personality is set in stone that we are naturally timid or impatient or depressed and can never change for the better.

This view is a misconception: in reality all things are in the nature of change, moment by moment all things change. Nothing is static and nothing possesses the nature of permanence. If we can understand how we, and the world we experience, come into being and disappear moment by moment we can use this wisdom to begin to take an active part in transforming our life. Beginning to glimpse the possibility that we actually create and shape the world according to our own level of wisdom/understanding is a very empowering experience.

At the moment it appears to us that we and the outside world are two separate phenomena when in reality our environment, our body, and even our sense of self/I are simply projections of our mind. We feel that we and the world around us definitely exist and that our senses are not fooling us! But this is not the case.

Dream of life

Buddha revealed this truth by likening everyday experience to a dream. In a dream everything seems real. We might dream that we are climbing a mountain, we can feel and hear the snow crunching beneath our feet, feel the cool wind or the warm sun on our face, if we look up we might see the top of this huge mountain far above us and beyond it the endless beautiful blue sky. In this dream you might be climbing with someone, a friend, and be talking about a dream that you had last night! Then when you wake up all these sensations and experiences that seemed so real have all gone. Where did they come from and where did they go to? They were simply a projection or creation of our subtle mind. They didn't exist in the way that they appeared, in the dream it all seemed very real but it was all just a creation of mind and an appearance to mind.

So it is with everyday life. People and places and all our experiences appear real but in reality they are simply mental projections from within our own mind, just like a dream!

This is a huge concept with many implications and opportunities for misunderstanding! Correctly understanding and experiencing this truth is the essence of the Buddhist path to enlightenment. The best way to really develop clear wisdom of what is being suggested here is to read books that deal specifically with this topic (like *Heart of Wisdom* by Geshe Kelsang Gyatso, Tharpa Publications) or to attend talks or classes given by a qualified teacher (see Appendix 4).

For now though simply contemplating that this truth might be the foundation or source of all life, the earth and planets, and all the myriad universes is enough! Second degree Reiki can help us to look at ourselves and the world around us in a new way. It can help us to consider that in one sense we are at the center of all things and that by learning to control and change our mind we can change everything.

This may seem like impossible fantasy but we know from experience that we all live in a slightly different world. We all perceive the external world in a slightly different way. Some mentally ill people perceive perfectly harmless things and environments as hellishly frightening simply because their mind perceives these things as so. Even our own view on the world changes according to our mood. We might wake up one morning feeling great, everything seems wonderful, colors seem brighter, people friendlier, we smile easily, the simplest things might cause us pleasure, then if we receive some bad news: our mind changes, we might feel depressed, and the whole world appears to darken.

Again this shows that as Buddha said "everything depends upon the mind." Ultimately we won't find the answers to the world's problems by going into outer space, or by mastering genetics or any other field of science. Our problem is not our job, relationship, house; our problem is our mind. If we can learn how to change our mind for the better regardless of external conditions we are well on the way to lasting happiness and through sharing our experience of this with others we are giving them something truly priceless, liberating, and meaningful.

Applying the techniques we learn in second degree Reiki in this way is a sign of great wisdom and maturity.

The meaning of symbols

> There is no spell more potent than that cast by mysterious symbols of which the meaning has been forgotten. Who can tell what ancient wisdom might be embodied in these enigmatic shapes and forms?
>
> E. H. Gombrich, *The Sense of Order*

This quote captures the thinking of many people in the West, especially those who have little experience or knowledge of spiritual paths. Many spiritual teachers and traditions have come to the West bringing with them wisdom gathered over thousands of years. Yet many scientists, anthropologists, and archaeologists think these are dead arts, and that the symbols that accompany them, their uses, and meanings have little or no place or value in the modern world. And yet this quote obviously shows a great intrigue and interest in such things, which is also the case with many Westerners.

Many, if not all, spiritual traditions use symbols in one form or another. The most famous of Christian symbols, the cross, carries an incredible depth of power and meaning for devoted

Christians. It is a sign of Christ's victory over death and the promise of everlasting life to those who follow his teachings and develop a living relationship with him as a spiritual guide. Many Christians wear this symbol, all churches contain it in many forms, it is a center or focal point for the whole tradition – a very simple but very potent and powerful symbol.

As mentioned, if you were not a Christian though and had never seen a cross before it would simply appear as two lines forming a cross. It would have no power and no meaning for you. This is a very interesting point then. Is the power that symbols possess simply projected on to them by the minds that perceive them? Does a cross have any power from its own side? This brings us back to the truth that "everything depends upon the mind."

How then can symbols help us and specifically how can the Reiki symbols assist and enhance our practice of healing and spiritual development? Well the mind works on many levels, the gross, obvious, or conscious mind that we are experiencing now and every waking moment sees the world in a very concrete two or three-dimensional way. However, there are many layers of consciousness within the mind, many subtle layers that we generally only experience whilst sleeping or dreaming. These layers of mind relate to the world in a very different way.

Our subtle or subconscious mind, the mind that manifests whilst we are dreaming, is generally not manifest throughout the day as we are so busy and preoccupied with the external world. If we were able to purify and then experience these subtler levels of mind and still remain conscious, as many advanced meditators and spiritual practitioners can do, we would understand, experience, and relate to others and the world around us in a very different way. We would begin to realize that our experiences in everyday life are very similar to what we normally experience whilst dreaming, that all phenomena are really just appearances to mind, or projections of the mind, as in a dream. For us at the moment we find this hard to believe simply because we are so used to relating to the external world as definitely "out there" – outside and separate from us.

If we could deeply understand our mind we would relate to the external world as a projection of the mind and see everything as a mirror or as a symbolic representation of ourselves. We can use external symbols that connect or help us to access or experience our subtle mind, so revealing this inner wisdom to the conscious mind. Once we begin to relate to the external world as a projection of our own mind or as a symbolic representation of our own good and not so good qualities this is a sign that we are really progressing well.

The following extract from *Reiki For Beginners* (published by Llewellyn) explains this in more detail:

> We can say that our body, environment, relationships, job, car, etc., are like reflections of our gross, subtle, and very subtle mind. Gross objects, like everyday solid forms, people, relationships, environments, etc. are like reflections of our gross mind; subtle objects, like those in dreams, are like reflections of our subtle mind; and very subtle objects, that are impossible for most people to perceive, are like reflections of our very subtle mind. We can interpret the subtle and very subtle mind as the subconscious mind or that part of our mind that we cannot consciously control or that we do not clearly "know." From early childhood and from generation to generation we have been taught to live in response to the external "real" world; we are unfamiliar or generally unaware of our internal nature and the problems and potential therein. So we cannot help but project ourselves, our faults and imperfections, onto the outside world and we do this so completely that we almost forget where we really come from.
>
> If we have external problems with health, finances, friendships, or anything else, this is like a bell ringing, a symbolic message saying that there is some part of us either mentally, emotionally, or spiritually that needs attention. At first this idea may seem

unusual but with experience we can begin to see clearly that our faults or imperfections are constantly being reflected or "given back" to us by our bodies, the environment, and our everyday experiences. Most people accept that if we suppress or over-indulge strong negative thoughts or emotions for a long time this can lead to physical or "external" health problems, harmful addictions, etc. Following on from this understanding if we ask ourselves, "What am I unhappy about?" "What problems do I have at the moment?" we can trace these outward manifestations back to some aspect of our inner nature that is not fully developed or in harmony with the whole.

For example, when people are lonely they can turn to food, drink, cigarettes, shopping, superficial relationships, etc. Consequently if we have problems/addictions in these areas it might be because we are lonely. If we can identify the true mental or emotional cause of the external problem we are half way to solving the issue. The other half of the answer is having the real desire to change, regain, and rebuild/develop that inner part of us that we have lost or abandoned and are presently looking to replace with some external comfort or support. In the case of loneliness we can try to release the need to gain happiness from others or external objects and develop an inner sense of acceptance, then contentment, and eventually deep peace and joy. This does not mean we have to abandon relationships or other physical pleasures, in fact releasing the "need" for these things actually allows us to gain greater enjoyment from them, our relationships become clearer, healthier, and more rewarding. It can take time to release our old habits, and create and feel deep contentment but it can be done if our wish to change becomes consistently stronger than our negative beliefs and habits. Reiki can help us greatly along this inner path.

On a less obvious or more subtle level, specific health problems can be symbolically related to specific causes in the mind. For example, we use our shoulders to carry heavy weights therefore shoulder problems can be related to carrying too much responsibility or not being responsible enough. Also our neck is very flexible and allows us to look in different directions, so neck problems can be related to rigid thinking or being too flexible by "giving in" to others. We use our eyes to see where we are going, so eye problems can be related to not wanting to see things as they really are or trying to hard to control things. We use our legs to move forward in life, so leg problems can be related to wanting to stay in a particular situation perhaps because it feels safe or striving too hard to achieve the wrong things. We can apply this line of thinking to any health problem, just think, "What is this problem telling me about myself?" "What does this issue represent symbolically?" Generally there are two extremes and a healthy middle way. If we sit and think about this quietly and honestly the answer will usually come simply and easily; we know ourselves better than we think! Don't make it complicated, just keep an open mind, remember all the answers are within you and if you don't feel ready or able to change you don't have to. You choose!

We can even apply this wisdom to apparently inanimate objects. For example, if your car battery is flat do you need more time to rest and recharge? If the front door to your house is jamming do you have difficulty letting people into your life or are you too open and accommodating? If you have a burst pipe or an electric bulb "goes," are you under too much pressure or do you always seek to avoid stressful situations for a quiet life? This may all seem a little "far-fetched" but with practice we can develop the wisdom to see ourselves everywhere and to use every situation as an opportunity to learn about our inner nature through its reflection in the external world. Obviously this way of looking at the world can also tell us what we are doing right! So if we are generally content, have good relationships, etc., this indicates that we are moving in the right direction.

Connecting with symbols

There are many esoteric symbols that spiritual practitioners use and have used in previous ages to access or manifest their own inner wisdom. Reiki practitioners have a special karmic connection with the Reiki symbols. We may have used this energy and symbols in previous lives so that we already have some subtle memories of their uses and power to help us. If we haven't used them previously then the symbols still have a special power to help us connect with our subtle levels of consciousness as during the Reiki attunements we receive a special blessing when the symbols themselves are transmitted or imprinted in the subtle mind. Then when we use them consciously we are directly working with our own subtle mind. It is then very easy for us to have spontaneous faith in their ability to help us as they are already part of us on some deep inner level.

Those symbols that we do not have a deep mental connection with will have little effect upon us unless we convince ourselves that they have great power from their own side to heal us. Often we project this power onto things and people subconsciously and then it appears to our conscious mind that these objects have great power from their own side. Some times this kind of "blind faith" can be very helpful in our spiritual development, especially if we realize when it is right to let our mind work in this way.

Buddhists use faith very successfully to propel them along the spiritual path although they know that eventually they will directly realize that even Buddhas do not exist inherently, like all phenomena they are simply appearances to mind like in a vivid dream! Buddha taught this truth to help us realize our own dream-like nature. To become a Buddha all we have to do is realize the nature/essence of our own mind.

Understanding that symbols only carry the power that we project onto them either consciously or subconsciously we can still regard them as tools for personal growth and spiritual development. We can still use them as if they are very powerful from their own side if this helps us in our healing or spiritual practice.

Characteristics of symbols

Second degree practitioners are often given a list of the characteristics of symbols. Sometimes the Reiki Master will explain these qualities immediately to the students and sometimes they are asked to take them away and consider their own explanation before returning to discuss their thoughts and ideas with the group.

Here is a typical list of the characteristics of symbols: they are applicable to all symbols but especially to the Reiki symbols. Some explanations are given after the list although sometimes it is better to see what they mean to you without being too influenced by others' thoughts. Some Masters regard this information as sacred and not to be discussed with those who do not have the second degree attunements. You can use your own discretion; basically universal truths are there for us all to benefit from, however it is unwise to talk about something you regard as precious and special with those who might create negative karma for themselves by deriding it or your efforts to appreciate it. If you are not clear about something relating to symbols or any aspect of second degree find a good Reiki Master and discuss it with her or him.

- Symbols are carriers of soul energy, they come from and return to the one source. (From a Buddhist perspective this one source is called "emptiness" or shunyata in sanskrit – see Heart of Wisdom by Geshe Kelsang Gyatso, Tharpa Publications.)
- Symbols are transformational, consciously and subconsciously.
- A symbol carries and possesses the vibration of what it is.
- A symbol is a key. A symbol is especially a key to the subtle mind.
- Symbols are a way to discover and access universal knowledge beyond the three dimensional world.

- Symbols take the individual from the particular to the universal.
- A symbol is a key to higher truth and what the nature of that truth is.
- Symbols return us to wholeness.
- Symbols integrate without interpreting.
- They are inclusive and expansive.
- Symbols center on unification and lead us to the power beyond the symbol.
- They convey life force energy, which supports, guides, and motivates us.
- Symbols open up and reveal deeper levels of understanding.

Sacred symbols as well as connecting the conscious mind with the subconscious also connect us with the divine. They are the energetic "bridge" that enables us to access divine blessings and levels of consciousness normally beyond the reach of ordinary minds. Because of this they are transformational. Each symbol has a specific use and purpose and a particular vibration of subtle life force energy.

Because we can use symbols as transformational tools and they enable us to access our inner wisdom and the natural wisdom of the cosmos they can be called keys. They have the power to unlock our potential for great happiness and wisdom.

This potential can only be accessed by learning to gradually abandon our sense of self-importance or individuality. Surrendering ourselves to the divine order of things, the expansion of happiness for all, might sound a little too weird or slavish, especially when we are talking about self-empowerment. But there is no contradiction and much benefit in letting go of our wish to control or manipulate the world as we would have it.

Ultimately we cannot deny that there is someone or something "up there" or within us that is great, wise, and infinitely good. The longer we separate ourselves from this special spiritual consciousness the longer it will take for our spiritual development. Communion with this limitless goodness is the key to inner transformation. One of the beauties of using symbols is that they are very experiential. The people who gain the most from using them are not necessarily those who have a good intellectual understanding but are simply willing to open their hearts and take the risk of being touched and transformed. Symbols help us to integrate divine consciousness into our lives on an experiential level without us necessarily having to intellectually interpret our experiences. This can help to keep our path spontaneous and alive instead of intellectual and dull. However, the intellect is vitally important to the path, we need it to map read! Then once you know the way, walk the path but regularly check you are still on the right path!

Our karma and the power behind the symbol create it. The Reiki symbols can lead us to the source of the power behind the symbol by stripping away the layers of wrong view or misconception within our own mind. The closer we approach this truth the more we come to understand that we are the same nature as the power behind the symbol and that the symbol is part of or simply a projection of our own higher self or divinity reaching out to us from deep within.

Receiving the Reiki symbols

The Reiki symbols themselves have individual and special meanings and these are explained in the next chapter. They each also possess the characteristics mentioned above, as do many other esoteric symbols, which we can learn to use in the same way. We can also learn to create our own symbols that have particular power and meaning for us and create new symbols for our Reiki patients to help their healing process. We can write them down and give them to our patients to look at, hold, or visualize once or twice a day. The possibilities and creative healing potential are limitless, all we need is a little imagination, confidence, and experience. We can have great fun learning these new techniques and sharing our insights with Reiki friends.

Receiving the symbols and their meaning from your Master in the second degree class is a very special experience. Because they are already a part of you, as a result of the attunement process, you may feel some kind of close connection with them. Many people feel that they have seen them before or that they remind them of something. Some people have a strong emotional response and feel very happy or deeply touched and privileged to receive them. Also some people might experience an emotional release like crying as some kind of inner healing is triggered.

Generally the whole second degree experience is very healing on many levels. It can feel very empowering as we are taught how to use the symbols for healing, spiritual growth, and in everyday situations. We might feel that we are moving closer to an understanding or inner knowing of what Reiki is and where it comes from. We might feel that we are becoming more like Reiki and that Reiki is absorbing into our daily activities and revealing many truths and opportunities for personal understanding and inner growth.

Other well-known symbols

We might only think that symbols were used in ancient times but nowadays we are actually surrounded by symbols. All our road signs are symbols, all company logos are symbols, flags are symbols, and there are countless other examples. There well known symbols that represent peace or power, good or evil. Even these type of "ordinary" symbols can be quite powerful. For example a "no entry" sign or a "one way" sign on a road has very powerful implications. If we try to do the opposite of what these symbols represent we may experience worry or guilt and fear of being caught. The fact that such a simple sign can have a powerful effect on the mind indicates how influenced we are by symbols. Company logos or designer labels can cause envy, pride, hatred, solidarity, etc. The essence of what the company or organization represents or stands for is encapsulated in the symbol. Or more accurately we project these qualities on to the symbol, which gives it the power to affect us!

Here are some well-known symbols used by different religions. To the follower of a particular religion the individual symbol has great personal meaning and can induce a deep emotional response. To a follower of another religion they can also induce a good response, no response at all, or even negative feelings. Again it all depends upon the mind.

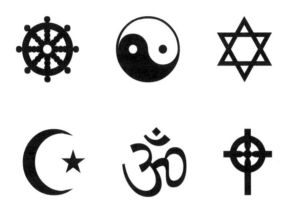

The sacred spiral
Some symbols have very special qualities. Although we can say that the power of any symbol ultimately comes from the mind that beholds it some symbols do seem to have a special place in the great scheme of things.

How is it possible for the same symbols to be used by different cultures, which developed thousands of years ago and thousands of miles apart, without any physical contact or awareness of the existence of each other? There are only a few symbols that fall into this special category like the "eternal knot," maze, or labyrinth.

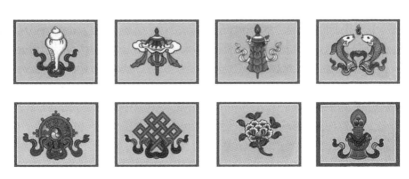

8 Auspicious symbols – (top row) right-coiled white conch, precious umbrella, victory banner, golden fish, (bottom row) dharma wheel, auspicious drawing, lotus flower and vase of treasure

The most commonly found symbol found within many ancient cultures is the simple spiral or as many people like to call it the "sacred spiral." It is found in the Egyptian, Celtic, Buddhist, Hindu, Christian, Aztec, and Muslim traditions and many others. It is found in ancient forms of sculpture, architecture, painting, pottery, rock carvings, as a metaphor in literature and in ancient spiritual texts. It is still used extensively today in many ways, if we look around us we will start to see it appearing in our lives. It is a common icon or graphic design and frequently used in sayings like, "on an upward spiral," or "spiraling out of control." Why should this be and what meaning or power does this symbol possess?

The spiral appears frequently in nature; grass and some plants and trees grow in a spiral, the rings of a tree are similar to a spiral, DNA has a spiral structure, whirl pools, tornadoes, and twisters form spirals. The cross-section shape of a breaking wave, many shells, and other natural objects form spirals. Also the circular motion represented by a spiral is mirrored in many things like the spinning of the planets on their axis and around the sun, even the tendency for history to repeat itself or for individuals to have repetitive behavior.

The major difference between the circle and the spiral is that the spiral represents evolution or regression, whereas the circle represents repetition. However, they are still closely linked and in terms of personal growth, one often becomes the other as we evolve spiritually in stages of slow or rapid growth (the upward spiral) between plateaus of stasis (the constant circle).

The famous Tibetan Buddhist Wheel of Life (page 33) is a symbolic map of cyclic existence showing the constant cycle of birth, ageing, sickness, and death that all beings are constantly experiencing and repeating. Those who have made the effort to complete the spiritual spiral to enlightenment have left this cycle forever and experience only peace and happiness. They also have the ability to lead others to the same state. In a way the spiral also represents the wheel of life. It can represent the upward spiral of the spiritual practitioner toward her or his ultimate goal or in reverse it can represent the spiral downward of the selfish mind. (See Joyful Path of Good Fortune by Geshe Kelsang Gyatso, Tharpa Publications for a complete explanation of the Wheel of Life, line drawing p33)

The way we view such a simple but powerful symbol and what we believe its qualities to be will dictate the degree of benefit we derive from it. Many people know nowadays that one of the Reiki symbols is based on the sacred spiral although the name or mantra associated with it and the way it is drawn or used is quite distinct. The qualities of this symbol and how it is used are given in the next chapter.

Symbols in everyday life

As mentioned before, we can see the external world as a symbolic representation of our mind. The way things appear and occur on the outside are a reflection of what we cannot see on the inside. The fact that we live in a universe with an infinite amount of outer space is very symbolic of our lack of inner space or inner awareness. Mankind has been preoccupied with conquering the external world since the beginning of time. Yet still we are not satisfied. No doubt this will continue, no doubt men and women will go to Mars then beyond, then beyond that. But still we are and will be experiencing the same personal problems that the very first human beings experienced.

External problems, like not always getting what we want, losing what we have, sickness, ageing, and finally death, these problems will never be overcome by external means. Women and men far into the future will also experience inner problems like anger, impatience, sadness, jealousy, guilt, grief, etc. No matter how far we "progress" or "advance" externally and no matter how good our external conditions become we will never find any lasting happiness unless we look within. We need to make the leap in consciousness from the external to the internal world, from outer development to inner development.

Because our outer world is a symbolic reflection of our inner world if we develop a peaceful and happy mind we will live in a peaceful and happy world. It really is that simple. Contentment is the key to lasting happiness. We will never fulfill all our desires in the external world, and trying to do so just reinforces the habit of looking for happiness outside of ourselves. The essence of the spiritual path is happiness from within for ourselves and others. Symbols are keys that can help us abandon negative habits and harmful views and develop the minds that lead to inner peace, self-acceptance, contentment, and the special minds of wisdom and compassion.

In everyday life if we are experiencing regular anger, impatience, discontentment, and so on these are the very obvious symbols telling us that we need to develop patience, contentment, balanced love, etc. We develop these qualities simply by changing the mind through prayer, meditation, Reiki, and/or simply developing the wish to change and then making the effort every day to do so. The mind is not made of stone; Buddha defined the qualities of consciousness as simply clear and cognizing (or understanding and experiencing). If we are grasping at our character or nature as truly lacking in confidence or truly impatient, or truly arrogant, this is only a simple mental projection. Given time and effort we can transform in to something truly special!

Ancient symbols

There is no doubt that people in ancient cultures such as the American Indians, Aborigines, Celts, Aztecs, etc. held a special regard for and understood the language of symbols. They would have been interwoven into everyday life and since life and death in those days walked hand in hand the symbols they used would have special significance in the associated rituals linking this world with the next, the rituals regarding the turning of the seasons, the planting and harvesting of crops, and so on. Because life was fragile and people were vulnerable these things had great meaning; nowadays we are encouraged not to think about death and the fragility of life and yet our own death might only be a breath away. If we think about the presence and possibility of death on a regular basis this will encourage us to make the most of our life and to try and derive some meaning from it. To the peoples of the ancient cultures their symbols were "alive," "energetic," and vibrating with life and to them they held great meaning and power.

If we can view and experience the Reiki symbols with a similar kind of reverence and joy, learning to play with them and allowing them to touch us deeply, then we will have much fun and gain great insight into ourselves and the meaning of our precious human life. The Reiki symbols can help to propel us swiftly and safely along our path, whatever form that might take.

5

The power symbol

Second degree Reiki is usually taught over two evenings or one weekend.

As with first degree we do not need to worry whether second degree will work for us; it will. Even if we do not experience any special feeling during the course or attunements we have still definitely received what we need and the symbols will begin to work their magic for us. Some Reiki Masters say that they prefer their students not to expect any wonderful experiences during the course but simply to come with the wish to start a deeper long-term relationship with Reiki based on their experience of first degree.

One of the special qualities of Reiki healing is that it is mainly spontaneous and natural. We do not have to make any great personal sacrifices or effort to receive this special healing ability. We do not need to complete long arduous spiritual retreats, go on special pilgrimages, or seek out elusive holy beings.

Even the founder of Reiki, Dr. Usui said in an interview that,

> I was not initiated in to this method by anyone in the universe. I also did not have to make any special efforts to achieve supernormal healing powers. While I fasted, I touched an intense energy in a mysterious manner, I was inspired (attuned/empowered). As

in a coincidence, it became clear to me that I had been given the spiritual art of healing. Although I am the founder of this method, I find it hard to explain all of this more precisely.

Source: Reiki, The Legacy of Dr. Usui, by Frank
Arjara Petter, Lotus Light Publishing.

So we can see that Reiki is a very simple and natural phenomenon and it is worth remembering this when learning to use the symbols. Do not overcomplicate things; the techniques for using the symbols are simple and aimed at being useful in everyday life, which is where they will be most effective. If we are not happy with the idea of using symbols, perhaps because it does not fit in with our religious beliefs, we do not need to use them. We can simply take the attunements in order to benefit from the higher or purer energy and we can always use the symbols later in life if we wish.

Second degree do's and don'ts

Your own Reiki Master will give you certain guidelines on how to live your life with second degree Reiki based on what their Master told them and their own experience. Generally though it is requested that the Reiki students do not show the symbols or give the names of them or how to use the symbols to non-second degree people. Why the secrecy? Well it is not really secrecy, more sacredness, keeping things special and having respect for these special methods of healing. This helps us to keep a pure view of Reiki and therefore a clearer, purer, stronger link with higher Reiki, which is what we need to maintain in order to move along the path more swiftly. If we regard Reiki as a very common phenomenon, and not very special, we may not derive the same level of benefit from it as someone who regards it as special and sacred.

If second degree is being taught over two evenings one attunement is generally given on the first night followed by the Master showing the three symbols to the students. The students copy and write each symbol and the name of the symbol as the Master draws them. This can take a little time as one or two are fairly complex. We have to learn how to write or draw them correctly and we need over the following hours or days to memorize them and the names completely before destroying any trace of the written symbols. We might think this is pointless nowadays as the symbols have been printed in books and on the Internet. It is up to you and your Master to decide what is true to the essence of Reiki for that is what will bring you both the most benefit in the long run. If Dr. Usui expected high standards from his students he did this for a good reason, for their benefit not his own. If we disregard the symbols and sacred methods that he taught are we practicing Reiki or just a shadow of Reiki?

Generally on the second day or evening the students are taught how to use the symbols and some Masters like to give a second attunement although this is not always required. Also, some Masters like to have another revision session about two weeks later in order for students to ask questions and share experiences. It is also common nowadays for second degree students to do a certain number of absentee treatments before the Master feels they are fully qualified. There is no requirement, as with first degree, for the student to give themselves treatments for twenty one or thirty days but again this can be of great benefit. I would definitely recommend at least a seven-day self-treatment period and then maybe a seven-day period for treating others either hands on using the symbols or absentee. Again these treatments can be half the length of first degree treatments if you wish. An absentee treatment is even quicker as explained later.

Introduction to the symbols

So now we can look at the symbols individually and discuss their various uses, meanings, and purposes. Then later on we can examine the different ways we can use these symbols to enhance our use and experience of Reiki. Since most of the people who will read this text will have some experience of Reiki, or at least a wish to know more about it, revealing the following information, without showing the symbols or their names, will be helpful especially if we can maintain a wish to regard this as sacred Reiki information. This information though will not be of much use to us if we do not receive the attunements and complete the full course with a qualified Reiki Master (unless we wish to learn to use symbols to heal without Reiki) and we could never "successfully" use this information for negative purposes as the nature of Reiki is simply to help others. We will look at the first Reiki symbol in this chapter as it is the most commonly used and forms the basis for using the other symbols. The second and third Reiki symbols are discussed in the following chapter.

The first symbol – the power symbol

Your Master will give you the name or mantra of this symbol and show you how to draw it correctly. The translation or meaning of the mantra is "to make straight or align." This is the symbol that in some ways resembles the sacred spiral so an explanation and understanding of that can help us to fully integrate the meaning of this symbol.

In Jill Purse's book *The Mystic Spiral* (Thames and Hudson) she says that the spiral tendency within each of us is the longing for and growth toward wholeness. Jill's book gives examples of how the spiral appears in many ancient cultures and its meaning and use in these traditions. There is a common link with most of these and it is to do with growth, evolution of the soul, spiritual communion with the divine, receiving blessings from above, and receiving energy from the Earth below (depending on the direction of the spiral, i.e. clockwise or anticlockwise).

From a Reiki perspective we can use this symbol to:

- Activate and empower other symbols
- Receive Reiki

- Send Reiki to others
- Accelerate or amplify the Reiki we are giving ourselves or sending to others
- Localize or emphasize Reiki healing in a particular part of the body
- Apply or send Reiki to a particular situation or mental/emotional problem
- Give Reiki to any inanimate object
- Use it with prayer or meditation, as a tool for inner healing or to encourage purer states of consciousness
- Give it as a blessing to others
- Allow it to work of its own free will through us in order to reach others
- Use it to manifest/attract things that we or others need to achieve any personal goal
- Empower any Reiki intention

Within the broad guidelines given below there are so many wonderful things we can do, this is such a useful symbol. We can use it in very mundane or ordinary ways to help us find a parking space or a lost object or we can use in a very powerful and altruistic way to send a special blessing to a homeless person or a humanitarian disaster that we hear about anywhere in the world.

This symbol works quickly, swiftly, deeply, and powerfully. We can use it daily and as often as we like. Play with it, work with it, experiment, allow it to work through you in the same way that Reiki does.

Visualize it coming down from above and working through your body and mind. Draw it in the air and walk through it. Draw it in the air over the front of your house, over your car, over your children and loved ones. Walk the symbol in a field then go and sit in the center of it and ask Reiki to bless your body and mind. We need to be creative and open to blessings to get the most from symbols. Try to weave it into your daily life so that you develop a really close relationship with it. This close relationship might happen quite quickly and you might feel like this symbol and the other Reiki symbols and the essence of the loving power behind them has always been there waiting for you to get to this point in your life, almost like a homecoming.

Special qualities

We say that this symbol has the power to "make straight" or "align" because it has! It has the power to align us with the "greatest good," the love or intentions of God, Buddha, the Divine, or whatever we call the greatest good. This symbol is like a key to receiving blessings, inspiration, inner and outer healing directly from the source of such things whenever we or others need it. It is like a direct line to God or Reiki! This symbol has the power to bestow harmony and peace, to bring clarity and understanding, and to promote minds that accord or are "in line" with the expansion of supreme happiness and good fortune for all living beings. In its purest state we can experience it as a subtle and sublime blessing or communion with all that is good and wise. Amazingly though this is also a very practical symbol! We can use it every day in many situations and for many purposes.

If we have completed first degree Reiki we will have a good knowledge of how to use Reiki by setting our intent for a particular purpose. We will probably also be aware that for our wishes or intentions to be truly beneficial they need to be for the "greatest good" for ourselves and others.

One of the main uses of the power symbol is that we can use it to wisely empower or amplify our abilities to fulfill our wishes or intentions. Simply by following the simple instructions given in the next chapter we can activate this symbol, access the special energy that is locked within it, and use this for whatever good purpose we wish. We do need to check our motivation regularly to make sure we are acting with the welfare of others and the "greatest good" in mind! We will look at the many ways we can use this symbol on a daily basis below. Experienced Reiki practitioners sometimes find that they use this symbol so much, as it is so useful, that they occasionally become too familiar with it or take it for granted. It is worth reminding yourself from time to time that this is a sacred or holy symbol and that our relationship with it should mainly remain on that basis. If we stop respecting it or gradually begin to use it for selfish gain it will begin to lose its power to empower our experience of Reiki.

As with the sacred or mystic spiral the power symbol can take us higher in our "spiral like" spiritual progress. It has the power to link or connect us to a very pure consciousness or energy and then encourages us to become more like this ourselves. Since our mind simply works through familiarity if we try to associate or mix our minds with this pure energy on a daily basis we cannot help becoming more like it ourselves. Just in the same way that if we spend too much time with those of a negative disposition we are more likely to develop negative tendencies. The more we use any of the Reiki symbols with a pure motivation the more we become familiar with the qualities of mind that they represent, the place where they originally arose from, and the same place within ourselves that they are leading us to.

The first symbol is called the power symbol simply because it gives our Reiki practice more power, not because it makes us more powerful. In fact as we progress along the Reiki path we actually become less powerful in the conventional sense of the word. This is a kind of process that has been described in many spiritual traditions as "surrendering." This is a gradual process of surrendering the self or abandoning selfishness. The power or intensity of higher Reiki serves to purify negative habits, ignorance, pride, laziness, impatience, attachment, and so on. This process is usually quite gentle in the same way that the heat of the spring sun melts the frozen winter wasteland and encourages the shoots of new healthy growth. Occasionally though it can also be quite swift and powerful like a raging forest fire! But we can develop the qualities to deal with such swift growth and after a little experience and given a little confidence we can even look forward to the thrill of it!

At the moment our mind is like a glass of muddy water. Sometimes it feels like our character or nature is truly shy, weak, selfish, proud, arrogant, etc. The mud is like our negative thoughts and emotions. As with the mind, if we filter and purify the water we will see that our essence is completely pure. Through purifying or realizing the nature of our mind we will directly see our true nature, which is still pristine, sublime, pure, and radiant. But we need to be realistic, it will take time to make significant progress, so try hard, work steadily, and be patient!

Specific uses for the power symbol

The following examples of the various ways we can use the power symbol are again mainly for second degree students only and we should regard all of this information as special and use it with a good motivation and respect for Reiki.

Empowering other symbols

If we are interested in using symbols in our spiritual growth then the first Reiki symbol, the Power Symbol, is indispensable. To use it to empower or breathe life into non-Reiki symbols we simply create a symbol sandwich! We follow the instructions given in the next chapter for creating and empowering the power symbol then we draw or imagine the non-Reiki symbol. Then we repeat the process of creating another power symbol so that the non-Reiki symbol is sandwiched between the two power symbols.

If we are simply meditating or visualizing the symbols we do not have to have a clear picture in our mind of all three symbols. We begin by setting our intention clearly. For example, if you are a Christian and you want to deepen your relationship with Jesus and

God you might choose to use the cross as a symbol of meditation. So you set an intention like "I would like to deepen my relationship with God and develop the Christian qualities of faith and kindness toward others." Then you activate the power symbol and meditate on it for a while, then you visualize the cross briefly and again activate another power symbol and then your proper meditation or prayer session can begin.

There are many powerful symbols in the universe and we should try to seek out those that have some meaning for us. We can use a picture of an enlightened being, like Buddha, as a symbol for meditation and personal growth. Again we would create and empower the power symbol as explained in the next chapter, briefly visualize Buddha or simply look at a picture or statue then create another power symbol and return to the visualization or simply meditate on the wish to develop similar qualities to an enlightened being. A powerful addition to this meditation is to imagine white light rays coming from the heart of the Buddha and filling our body and mind; we try to feel as if all our stress and negativity are melting into this light and our body and mind are becoming light, peaceful, and completely relaxed. We can even imagine that our body and mind completely melt in to this light and we become "one" nature.

Another meditation, once we have relaxed the body and mind, is to imagine deep down in our mind at the very center of our being is a spark of light. This spark is our Buddha nature or the seed of our own future enlightenment. Again we can imagine light rays coming from the heart of Buddha and filling our body and mind. But this time we focus on the spark of light in the depths of our soul. We try to feel as if it begins to gradually become brighter and brighter. Again as this inner light starts to shine from within we imagine all our stress and worries and any sickness begin to melt into this light and our body and mind become light and relaxed. We try to feel that the nature of this inner light is all good qualities like wisdom, love, compassion, patience, giving, etc. Then we can simply meditate on this experience of inner light for as long as we wish. This is a very simple but very powerful meditation, as we are meditating on or trying to realize/experience our true nature, if we can do it for a short time each day for a few weeks or months this will bring great inner peace and space into our lives. Also don't worry if you cannot visualize easily as this is not too important, we just need to feel or believe with a light and relaxed mind that it is actually happening, this is the key to successful meditation.

Using the power symbol like this is a way of inviting blessings or positive energy from above and asking Reiki to empower our meditation or help us to develop good qualities.

Another well-known transformational symbol is the Egyptian Ankh. It is similar to a cross but also like a man with outstretched arms. Again this is a good symbol for developing our spiritual side especially if our motivation is pure. We could draw and empower the Reiki power symbol over our forehead or third eye, then draw the Ankh in the same place and about the same size, then repeat the power symbol. We then visualize the Ankh in our mind's eye and see what happens! This is a very simple but special way to meditate on any transformational symbol and especially the Reiki symbols whilst we are actually giving or receiving Reiki. If we are uncomfortable with the idea of using symbols that are not part of our own religion or culture it can be helpful to imagine that they all come from the same "good" place, which simply manifests them in different cultures according to what different people can relate to.

We really need to experiment with different ideas and ways of using symbols. We can create our own symbols simply by spending some time "doodling" with pen and paper, or we can draw symbols that we know and adjust them to suit us. It is best to do this when you are relaxed or in a meditation or daydream kind of mood as our mind is more open to inspiration from "above" which is always helpful! The ones that will be most effective for us are those that make a deep impression on the mind, ones that make our heart react in a positive way. Also we may receive symbols in dreams.

However, this way of using symbols is wasted time if we are not using them with a good motivation. We shouldn't regard these techniques as simply an amusing or intriguing pastime or a way of "playing" at spirituality. These are spiritual tools for inner growth; if we disrespect them we are missing a special opportunity to really move along our inner path, then we may not have this opportunity again for a long time.

Receiving and sending Reiki

The power symbol gives us the opportunity to send second degree Reiki energy easily and quickly to any situation. If we see someone homeless on the street, someone obviously depressed or upset, someone physically or emotionally injured or in any negative situation then we can send these people Reiki to help them. We can do the same for people we read about or hear about on the radio or TV. This symbol works powerfully and quickly to help people in physical or mental distress or just in need of a little inspiration or love. Generally as you will see in the next chapter it helps if we can physically see the person or have a picture but if we just hear about someone's misfortune on the radio we can still use this symbol as the most important thing is simply intention: energy follows intention.

Again as you will read in the next chapter we mentally draw the symbol above the person's head before activating it. We don't need to move or say anything out loud, so no one needs to know we are doing anything and often if we keep our healing actions to ourselves they become more powerful causes for our own and others' future happiness. We can set a mental intention before doing this like "may this person experience relief from their problems swiftly and easily" or we can be very specific like "may that lost dog find a loving home." If we do not know what will be the best for someone we can put our intention in the hands of Reiki and think "may this person receive Reiki blessings for their greatest good."

When we become experienced we might feel comfortable simply looking at someone and "knowing" that Reiki will give them what they need, then we use the symbol. Or we might find the symbol seems to draw itself as soon as we experience a sense of compassion toward another.

We can "zap" a crowd of people with a power symbol, a neighborhood, a city, a whole nation, or the entire world population! Intention is everything. If we are in a crowd, like at a football match or in a theatre or shopping in a busy place, we can think, "may all these people be blessed and find lasting happiness and freedom from all problems." Then we can mentally draw the power symbol over the whole crowd and activate it and/or we can imagine that each person receives a power symbol over their head perhaps all raining down from a very big power symbol. Really whatever feels good is the correct method, as long as we have a good, clear motivation and draw and activate the power symbol correctly it will work for their highest good.

To "zap" a country or the whole world, simply visualize the planet or the outline of the country perhaps using a map if you are not familiar with it, set your intention, draw and activate the symbol.

You are probably beginning to see now how incredibly powerful, versatile, and useful this symbol can be. It is really the powerhouse of second degree Reiki. Without it the other symbols would not be so useful. So it really is important if we want to make the most of second degree to use this symbol in many different ways and get to know it really well.

The power symbol in healing

As well as using the power symbol to help others we need to use it for our own healing and inner growth. This is a very powerful healing symbol and there are many ways we can use it both in formal treatments and everyday life. The only limit is our imagination and intention.

One of the most common ways to use this symbol in a formal treatment either for yourself or when treating others is to draw and activate the symbol over your palm chakras, then over your head, third eye (forehead), throat, and heart chakra. Some people like to carry on down the body to cover all the chakras. This might be especially helpful if you intend to concentrate Reiki in these areas. We do not always have to physically draw the symbols, we can just imagine them appearing or drawing themselves and then we can silently activate them according to the instructions in the next chapter. This symbol is perfect for concentrating healing energy in a particular part of the body. If we are working through the normal twelve positions when we arrive in an area that we feel needs an extra boost we draw or imagine the symbol appearing over that area and activate it, then carry on with the normal treatment. Another alternative it to redraw and activate power symbols on the palms and then a third over the area to be treated. However, breaking contact with the body during the treatment is not generally a good thing.

Some people like to imagine countless tiny golden power symbols pervading every cell of the body or just the area where we want to concentrate Reiki. We can imagine the power symbol in different colors according to the nearest chakra. We can imagine that the whole treatment room is full of floating power symbols of different sizes and colors or we can visualize one golden power symbol over the patient's head and a constant stream of smaller ones coming out of this and dissolving into the patient's body purifying any sickness or illness.

We can imagine one huge power symbol over our house or in the healing room before a treatment. We can draw one over the treatment couch in between treatments to cleanse the area. If we are preparing a natural remedy (like Bach Flower) we can use the power symbol to empower it with Reiki. We can use the power symbol on drinks or food for healing purposes. As always set a good motivation or intention, draw or visualize the symbol over the cup or plate, activate the symbol, and then if you have time place your hands round the cup or over the plate and give the food or drink a few minutes hands-on Reiki. This also works especially well with spring or filtered water.

If we want to concentrate Reiki on a particular aspect of the mind we need to use the second Reiki symbol for mental and emotional healing, which is introduced later. Even the second Reiki symbol cannot be used without the first, as mentioned above to use it most effectively we need to "sandwich" it between two power symbols, this technique is explained later.

There are really so many ways we can use the power symbol and so many ways we can bring more Reiki into the world swiftly and powerfully. Some people like to use complicated and colorful visualizations and some people simply prefer to set a simple intent, draw and activate the symbol over the crown chakra and leave it at that. Both are valid methods; we simply need to play with various ways until we discover our own preferences.

One word of advice, though: it can be helpful sometimes just to keep things simple and let Reiki and the symbols speak to you, work through you, and do the work for you. Listening to and experiencing what Reiki has to offer us is priceless. If our mind is always trying to direct Reiki this way and that and using too many wild visualizations we will never hear what Reiki has to say. Reiki has a subtle, quiet voice. Inner listening and being is a fine art that takes years of humble practice to master. True mastery comes through complete service to God/Buddha and to others and to our own inner potential. We can find lasting happiness and make swift progress toward enlightenment simply by losing our "self" in cherishing others.

The power symbol for spiritual growth

As mentioned earlier the power symbol comes from and can lead us to the divine. There are many mundane ways we can use this symbol to manifest our goals, like finding a parking space in a busy street, attracting wealth, a compatible partner and so on. It is fine for us to do this if we have a good motivation. But the real value of this symbol is its powerful spiritual simplicity and purity.

We can use this symbol in meditation in many ways and again we need to experiment and find ways that work well for us. One simple yet powerful way is to draw and activate the symbol over the palms and upper chakras, then over each wall of the room and on your seat or meditation cushion. Once you are seated, set an intention like, "through the blessings of this sacred symbol may I become whole, healthy, and happy and may my life become truly meaningful." Then again we can draw or visualize the symbol over our crown chakra, third eye, throat, and heart.

We can then meditate on various things like a constant stream of golden light coming from above and blessing our body and mind. Or we can gently repeat the name of the power symbol like a mantra. Or we can simply concentrate on the wish to become a more kind and compassionate person, more Christ or Buddha like.

We can also use well-known mantras like "OM MANE PAME HUM": this mantra is great for developing compassion and kindness, at the same time we can imagine our body and mind being blessed with white light. Another simpler mantra is "OM AH HUM": this is the mantra of all enlightened beings and is very blessed. The meditation we can do with this mantra is very profound and powerful yet simple, it is explained in Appendix 1.

Using the power symbol on a daily basis

As mentioned there are countless ways we can use this symbol to help others and to make our own life more "in tune" with reality. When we send or give the symbol to others either secretly or openly to another Reiki person we are asking the universe or God to bless them for their greatest good. Of course we can set specific intentions although the symbol like Reiki will only ever work for our and others' greatest good.

We know that this is a sacred esoteric symbol and that similar spiral-like symbols have been used for spiritual purposes for a long time. So how is it that we can use this symbol for general mundane purposes? Well, if we are generally living our lives with a good heart and we want to ripen our spiritual potential and make our lives meaningful there is no reason why we shouldn't use the symbol as part of this journey. The symbol can help in many ways to make our path smooth and swift both physically and mentally. We can use it to make our lives a little simpler so we can find the right conditions and time to concentrate on what really matters.

If we are moving house or looking for a new car, looking for a new job, or wondering how to use our retirement, looking for somewhere to go on holiday, or stuck in a traffic jamb, these are all situations where we can use the symbol to remove obstacles and bring clarity swiftly. Also things like finding a lost object, mending a broken watch or computer, baking a cake, or more serious things like healing difficult relationships are things that respond well to the power symbol. As mentioned we bring the object, situation, or person to mind, set our intent mentally (or verbally if appropriate), draw the symbol and activate it. If we can see the object directly, and we are alone, we can physically draw and activate the symbol then apply a few minutes' hands on Reiki. If we are looking for a lost object, visualize it, set an intent like "may I find this object swiftly and easily," then mentally or physically draw the symbol and activate it.

Apart from the obvious techniques of drawing and activating the symbol there is no right or wrong way to use it. Different Masters teach different techniques according to what they have been taught and what they have found to be helpful. If we are sending or giving the symbol to a person or persons, for say a relationship problem, we would generally imagine the symbol over the head or forehead but other than that we can be creative or just trust the symbol. Often it is the heart area we need to concentrate on (not the physical heart but the spiritual heart, which is located in the center of the body at the level of the physical heart); this is the area within the body where our very subtle mind or soul is located. Interestingly it is also the area of the body that we relate to when we think or feel "I" or "me."

If we have difficulty visualizing the symbols this is not a problem. Some people prefer to work through feelings instead. This can be just as powerful, if not more so. We can just feel the presence of the symbol or the symbol's blessings, then try to visualize it as best we can (if it is not appropriate to draw it in the air) and activate it as usual. This can be a very intimate and profound way to use symbols and something that can really deepen our experience of Reiki's special blessings.

Whatever reason we use the symbol or whatever intentions we set if nothing happens or just the opposite happens we need to think again about our motivation and check that it is in accordance with the greatest good. Our own mind is a subtle object and quite difficult to see clearly; our own motivations can be clouded and tinged with selfishness even when we think we are being very altruistic. It can take years to really get to know our own mind so take your time and when things don't work out as you had hoped check your motivation and either try again, let it go, or adjust your intention. Again this is a learning process, part of the path, so try to keep a peaceful, light and happy mind and simply enjoy your journey.

A light mind

It is important to keep a light mind whatever kind of symbol work we are doing. Don't get too serious about things and have fun with working and discovering how to use the symbols. We are simply trying to increase our happiness and the happiness of others, nothing more and nothing less.

Try to avoid any sense of pride over others because you know the symbols and practice Reiki. Pride can be a very subtle state of selfishness so we need to be alert. One of the best ways to avert it is to regularly remind yourself that you are working for the benefit of others by spreading Reiki and helping to heal the world by increasing your own good qualities. If we think that we are in the service of others, as were Jesus and Buddha, then it is difficult to feel better or "higher" than others.

How to create and activate the power symbol

Once we have completed a second degree course and received the appropriate empowerments we will know how to create and activate the symbols. Some Masters teach slightly different methods and some will have added their own techniques, which they have found to be helpful; all methods will be effective if they don't differ too much from the original and if the Master is part of a direct lineage from Dr. Usui. Almost all Masters are part of a direct lineage these days since it was not long ago that Dr. Usui was alive. It takes hundreds of years for these types of lineages to degenerate so in terms of time we are still very close to Dr. Usui's influence or energy.

There are basically four guidelines for using the power symbol most effectively:

1. Intention
2. Creating the symbol
3. Activating the symbol
4. Dedication

Intention
First we set our intention. This can be simple and quick, for example when we want to use the power symbol as a blessing for someone in distress or someone we see on TV or for some ordinary purpose like giving Reiki to our food or drink. We can simply think one of the following intentions or something similar:

May this person receive a special Reiki blessing for their greatest/ highest good.

May this food be blessed for my good health.

We don't always have to set an intention, especially if we have confidence that Reiki will always work for the greatest good. We can just simply let the symbol do its thing although the advantage of making intentions and directing Reiki is that we create good karma, especially if our motivation is good. The more familiar we become at generating and setting good intentions the more "Reiki like" we will become.

Creating the symbol

Once we are happy with our intention we create the symbol simply by drawing it or visualizing it appearing in front or over the object or person we want it to help or bless. If we are directing Reiki specifically at one person we need to visualize them as best we can, assuming they are not present. Just a vague outline in your mind will do or actually just the intention is enough if you cannot see them in your mind's eye. Again feelings are very powerful in this process, feeling/believing that the other person is very present seems to create a connection or energetic "bridge" for Reiki to reach them. Saying their name three times can also help to create a connection. We can use a photograph as well to help with this process.

Draw the symbol (this might be in your mind's eye) so that it appears vertically above the head, on the forehead, or so that the lowest part of the symbol is just above the eyebrows. It can be a large or small symbol, whatever feels right to you, although there is a general feeling that larger symbols are more generous! If no one is with you or the person you are giving the symbol to is also a second degree practitioner you can physically draw the symbol in the air over and just in front of the area above the eyebrows. It is always nice to physically bring the symbols into being whenever you can, they seem to enjoy it too!

When you do draw them, use whichever hand feels most natural, keep the fingers and thumb gently together as you would in a Reiki treatment, using the fingertips as the drawing point. If you are drawing a very large symbol you could move your whole arm, rotating at the shoulder, and for a small one just the hand, rotating at the wrist. We need to practice this to find out what feels right and what Reiki likes!

If you are just visualizing the person you can still draw the symbol physically and at the same time see it in your mind's eye appearing over the person's head. You can of course just visualize this and after a while you might see symbols appearing in your mind's eye frequently above the heads of people you are with; this might happen even before you have the thought to use the symbol, again this is quite natural.

We can also send a symbol to many people at once. If we are walking down a busy street we can send a symbol to everyone we see, or all the people in your town, or to all the people involved in a difficult situation we hear about. It doesn't matter if you cannot visualize them clearly, the intention and our feeling/faith will direct the symbol. All we really have to do is draw it and activate it.

If you are using the symbol on an ordinary object like food or a car, again simply draw the symbol over the object, activate it, and enjoy the results. The power symbol fits nicely over a plate or in a glass if you draw it horizontally, again you can give your food or drink a few minutes' hands on Reiki as well. To find a lost object, bring the object to mind, set your intention, draw the symbol over it in your mind's eye, and activate it; soon the object will turn up or go to where it is needed more! This symbol is essentially a spiral of Reiki so we can also visualize it in a three-dimensional way as well with the first two lines forming the top or start of the symbol and the spiral moving toward or in to the object or person.

Activating the symbol
Once we have created or drawn the symbol we activate it simply

by saying the name of the symbol three times. We can just think it if there are other people present or say it out loud if we are alone. Then we can sit back and let the symbol work its magic. We can also take a more active role by using further visualizations like imagining the symbol working to bless the mind of someone. We can imagine that all their problems and difficulties are lessening and that they are happy and content. This may or may not actually happen, we do not know what others need and often it is better simply to "give it up" to Reiki and trust that they will be OK. However, meditations like these create really good karma and again we can dedicate or direct this positive energy for others. They also create very good tendencies like genuine compassion and inner strength, then eventually through training our mind in this way we will actually develop the power to directly release others from suffering.

We can use many symbols at once on one person. Just use one to start with as explained above, then imagine that whatever parts of the body are in need of healing receive a symbol or many symbols. Also different aspects of the mind or personality can be sent symbols, like the feminine and masculine sides, the inner child, the adult, the soul, and so on. Although generally these aspects can be healed more effectively with the second symbol for mental and emotional healing.

Dedication
As always when we perform any healing action or any good action like prayer or meditation or helping others or refraining from negative thoughts and deeds we need to dedicate the positive karma or energy that we have created. If we don't we can easily destroy it by developing a negative mind, then all our good efforts are wasted. If we mentally "bank" or direct our good karma for some good future purpose then we cannot destroy it and its power and potential actually increase with time. So we can simply think something like, "Through the force of this positive action may all living beings

find lasting happiness swiftly and easily and may my wisdom and compassion continually increase for their benefit." This is a very altruistic and unselfish intention and we may feel that we are giving away all our good karma, but, if our wishes are sincere, in actual fact we are increasing and multiplying it beyond our imagination. It is amazing that the more we think about the welfare of others the more we benefit! What more encouragement do we need to dedicate our lives to helping others by developing the minds of wisdom and compassion and sharing this great inner wealth with others.

So in conclusion use this symbol as often as you like but try to keep a special view or relationship with it.

6

Mental, emotional, and distant healing

The second symbol – the mental
and emotional healing symbol

As the name suggests the main function of this symbol is to heal the mind. The power symbol can also have a profound healing effect on the mental and emotional level but generally it is better to use the right tool for the right job.

We can broadly separate the mind into three levels of consciousness: the gross, subtle, and very subtle level. The gross level is the mind that we use on an everyday basis, i.e. the mind we are using now to read this book. Most people only experience the subtle mind when dreaming and the very subtle mind only manifests during deep sleep, also known as REM sleep. The subtle and very subtle minds also become manifest during the process of dying, as our mind dissolves inward and finally leaves the body to look for a new one!

Buddha said that "Everything depends upon the mind." Our mind colors and shapes the world we live in. It is quite correct to say that each of us lives in a slightly different universe; we all perceive the world around us in a slightly different way according to our mind. Obviously some of us, like animals and humans with severe mental health problems, perceive the world in a very different way than the rest of us. But even between people of like mind there are still many differing perceptions of reality.

Unfortunately only a very few people perceive the world or "reality" as it actually exists and because these beings are so highly evolved or enlightened we cannot see them or hear their words directly because our minds are still clouded with misconception. However, there is no doubt that if we have a sincere wish to develop spiritually then sooner or later we will meet a qualified spiritual teacher who can guide us along the path to enlightenment.

What relevance does this have to the mental and emotional healing symbol? Well, if everything depends upon the mind all we have to do to change our reality or solve our problems is to change our mind. We will never solve our problems or find real lasting happiness by manipulating and adjusting the external world. We will only find peace of mind by developing a peaceful mind.

The true nature of the mind is simply like a blank canvas and we can paint on it whatever beautiful experiences we wish to have. People with a generally angry mind have created an inner painting like a stormy sea or a raging fire, and the world for them is full of irritating people and difficult situations. People who look at the world with pessimism have created an inner picture full of dark colors and heavy shapes and the world for them is very bleak. Although the way these people view reality appears correct to them they do not realize that under all those layers of paint there is still a blank canvas.

We need to strip away these layers steadily and gradually then we can begin to understand that it is our own view that creates the world we experience. We can paint a new picture. Eventually our mind will become so pure and clear that we will only experience a pure world, good people, and a peaceful, happy mind; heaven on earth.

This is the essence and the goal of true mental and emotional healing and the ultimate meaning of the second symbol. Having established this, though, we need to learn how to use it on a practical day-to-day basis and how to treat people who are not interested in spiritual development but simply want relief from an unhappy or unpeaceful mind or simply physical healing. Of course it is impossible to separate the body, mind, and spirit (or very subtle mind) but on a practical level we have to learn to discriminate in order to communicate effectively with different people who ask us for Reiki.

The meaning of the symbol

Your Reiki teacher will introduce you to this symbol in the second degree class and show you how to draw or create it and then activate it for healing purposes or spiritual growth. They will also tell you the name or mantra of the symbol. Learning the name and how to draw the symbol is important and you will be expected to commit these things to memory and not to write them down or show them to non-second degree people; this is really important as mentioned in the last section on the power symbol.

The translation of the mantra reveals that the nature of this symbol is "the greatest peace" or it is sometimes translated more literally as "I have the key" or "key holder." This symbol is often described as the key and the guardian. The "key" aspect refers to its ability to unlock, reveal, and heal aspects of the mind that were previously hidden, i.e. parts of the subconscious or subtle mind. The "guardian" aspect reveals that this symbol has the power to protect us from negative influences and keep our own spiritual practice from degenerating if we use it regularly. The word mantra also means "mind protection."

The second Reiki symbol is also symbolically associated with the "dragon," a mythological creature regarded as a guardian of something precious. The treasure can be symbolic of the inner goal of spiritual realizations. We do not have to fight the dragon as is often believed; he is just the guardian and the guide helping us to develop the special inner qualities that will naturally reveal the inner treasures resulting from training and understanding our mind.

The subconscious is simply that which we are not consciously aware of. We may have mental and emotional problems/issues that we cannot clearly identify and may still be experiencing the conscious symptoms of them such as fatigue, irritability, physical stiffness, and so on. As soon as we can understand the inner problem on a conscious level and identify the causes, the symptoms generally become less troublesome and soon peace of mind is regained. This is one of the main benefits we can derive from using the mental and emotional healing symbol; it is like a mirror that reveals our inner world.

Like all Reiki symbols it is not a difficult symbol to use. Simplicity is the key to the whole system of Reiki healing. Although many books have been written on Reiki and many ideas developed to enhance the practice of Reiki, original Reiki, the essence of Reiki, is still very simple. We do not have to exert great effort to gain deep benefit from this method of healing and spiritual growth; once we have received the attunements and basic instructions we can practice with confidence without extensive study or clear understanding of what Reiki is or how it works. Books like this one can be helpful in advancing our understanding but they are not essential. We can often learn more simply by being in the presence of someone who is sincerely practicing Reiki with a good heart and genuinely "living" Reiki.

All our problems originate in the mind, so we can see the great value of a symbol that allows us to directly heal the inner causes of simple day-to-day problems and more deep-seated problems like serious illness, poverty, difficult relationships, and so on.

Greatest peace

As mentioned our very subtle or root mind is the very center of our being; perhaps some spiritual traditions would describe this as our soul. It is the "root" mind that goes from life to life, a mental continuum without a beginning or end. It is beyond the physical world, it is formless, and its essential nature is clarity and cognizing or "knowing." This pure clear consciousness is like a vast ocean and the thoughts and feelings and experiences of daily life are like the waves on the surface of the ocean. All our everyday thoughts and emotions arise from the very subtle mind before we experience them on a conscious or gross level. When we feel any strong emotions like fear, sadness, grief, anger, and so on, the surface of this inner ocean is stormy with huge waves and when we are peaceful, content, and happy this is like the surface of a calm ocean with a mirror-like quality.

When we fall asleep at night our gross or waking consciousness dissolves inward as we become sleepy and when we lose this normal consciousness and actually fall asleep we experience the subtler levels of mind like the dream state and the level of deep sleep, which is when the very subtle or root mind becomes manifest. This is why after a good night's sleep we feel so refreshed, as our conscious mind has returned "home" to the root mind and merged with this pure ocean of consciousness.

If we go without sleep for a few nights this can affect our mental and physical health so we can see how important this relationship is with our root mind, that special inner place that is the source of all.

In meditation we train to be able to manifest our very subtle mind whilst still remaining conscious, i.e. not falling asleep. When we are able to do this our whole life takes on a new meaning and perspective, we have more energy and clarity of mind, our sleep is less disturbed and we often need less sleep, our physical and mental health improves, and there are many others benefits apart from the special experience of meditation itself. Reiki can also bring these special benefits, especially the levels of second degree and higher.

As the Reiki we channel becomes purer, more subtle, and refined, the states of mind we experience on a daily basis also become more subtle. These subtler levels of mind reveal many truths about ourselves and others, we are given mental and spiritual clarity of mind, we begin to see things in a new light. If we can gain some knowledge and experience of meditation we can use this alongside our Reiki practice to bring wisdom to our experiences. This is priceless, as developing the wisdom to understand our Reiki experiences accelerates our spiritual growth and makes the path much smoother, more interesting and enjoyable. Also we cannot complete our path to spiritual perfection without a clear understanding of what the path is and how to walk it on a daily basis and without a spiritual guide we can easily lose our way.

One of the reasons why the mental and emotional Reiki symbol is called "Greatest Peace" is that it reduces distractions in the mind and calms negative or extreme mental and emotional states. By using second degree Reiki these violent mental waves gradually and gently dissolve back into the ocean of the mind from where they came, like waves dissolving back into the ocean so that our consciousness becomes peaceful again.

When we have a peaceful and happy mind and we are able to maintain it our body is less likely to become ill and if we develop illness it is more likely to pass quickly. Just having a peaceful, calm, and happy mind is a very special quality. We can be of great benefit to others if our own mind is generally calm and not severely affected by the changing fortunes of life. If we can learn to develop and maintain a mind like this we are doing something really special for our own family, friends, community, and even the whole world.

All the problems that arise in this world can be solved simply by each of us taking responsibility for the state of our mind and developing the wisdom and courage to look within. All wars arise from anger, stealing arises from the wish to possess what others have, all illness and natural disasters are the ripening karma of negative actions in previous lives, which again came from negative mental intentions. All the good things that happen in this world come from good or compassionate mental intentions. Only by understanding and transforming our mind can we find lasting peace and freedom from suffering. Without this simple wisdom we are lost.

If all the people in this world understood this and tried to keep a peaceful and happy mind and regarded the welfare of others to be really important there would be no basis for wars or famine or any kind of avoidable suffering. We could solve most of the world's problems in a few years. Then even when problems did arise we would still be able to maintain peace of mind and accept the situation instead of making things worse with worry and anxiety.

So on one level the essence of this symbol is that it simply grants us the ability to deepen our practice of inner contentment and peace of mind and share this with others. This may sound like a very simple or mundane spiritual goal. But really it is the very essence of the spiritual path. The spiritual path is simply the path to lasting happiness. We may not need to perform all kinds of complicated meditation practices to achieve this. Also as mentioned we are not looking for amazing spiritual experiences involving lights and colors, channeling angelic voices, levitating, clairvoyance, and so on. These practices or abilities can be great distractions to the pure spiritual practitioner and are actually byproducts of the spiritual path that will eventually come naturally. There are many people in this world who possess varying degrees of these special gifts but still experience the problems of an unhappy and unpeaceful mind.

There are fewer and fewer people in this world who are genuinely happy, peaceful, content, humble, considerate, compassionate, wise, friendly, patient, kind, and so on. There are even fewer people who value or who want to develop these qualities and yet they are the very qualities that bring us closer to God, closer to enlightenment, closer to pure and genuine lasting happiness.

The key to consciousness

The other main meaning of this symbol, "I have the key," indicates that it has the ability to help us transcend surface or normal consciousness and connect us with the subtler levels of our mind. We are being given a tool to unlock the door to the great inner treasure. This is the real Holy Grail, the source of all life and happiness. Locating and familiarizing ourselves with the special levels of subtle consciousness is a very natural process. We should never try to mentally force our mind to reveal its treasure but gently and steadily try to develop and allow these special minds to arise through the daily practice of Reiki and especially through using the symbols either as part of treating yourself and others or as tools for meditation.

This symbol allows us to unlock this special inner peace which, through regular practice, will gradually and naturally start to arise on a daily basis until eventually we feel blessed, peaceful, relaxed, and happy all the time. Through training our mind in this way we can even learn to retain this special way of "being" in difficult and challenging situations. Then whatever eventualities arise we can remain calm and content knowing that we have found lasting happiness from within and it will never desert us because it is our own source or root of existence which we can never be parted from.

Having this deep and stable happiness also, and perhaps most importantly, puts us in the position of being of the greatest benefit to others. At the very least we become a calm and stabilizing influence on others and at best we can share this inner peace and contentment with others by giving or teaching them Reiki or simple meditation techniques to help them control their own mind and develop lasting happiness from within.

Breaking the cycle

One of the most remarkable qualities of this symbol is that it allows us to break cycles of repetitive mental and emotional behavior, either our own or those of people to whom we are giving Reiki. These repetitive behavior patterns can be very gross and obvious such as drug, alcohol, or nicotine dependence or more subtle like stress at work, damaging relationships, inability to express or share feelings, and so on. As second degree practitioners we have a great chance to over come and heal these issues. However, the degree to which we can help non-Reiki patients also depends on their wish to change. Sometimes we may put a lot of time and effort into helping a patient who is only partly willing to change; this is never wasted energy as we will have definitely helped to create some positive potential in the mind for future healing. But we need to be aware that patients who have a genuine wish to "move on" should get some degree of priority. Everyone's time for healing will come, maybe not in this life, but it will come.

Reiki has the ability to alleviate and sometimes solve these problems without the use of symbols; also we might be a second degree practitioner but do not generally use the symbols yet we find we are able to help people with these types of problems. The symbols are simply an additional way we can approach these problems. The second Reiki symbol is especially helpful in any situation that requires mental and emotional healing. Since all our problems, whether physical, mental, or environmental, have their cause and potential cure within the mind we can see that this symbol should have a special place in our daily practice.

Imagine your mind like a three-dimensional grid of lines, where each line crosses another there is a little knot with some knots being small and easily undone and others being deeply tangled and tied tight. These knots represent things like negative thought patterns, repetitive behavior, guilt, painful memories, etc. Each time we allow our mind to be negative or compulsively repeat the same mistake or negative action or worry about the future or dwell on past pain we are tying some of these knots tighter. The more we do this the harder it will be to untie them and the more we are likely to continue repeating this behavior. If we don't make the effort to break these patterns they will bring us great stress, pain, and depression in the future. However, if we have faith, a strong and continuous wish, and apply regular and confident effort there is nothing to stop us completely removing all these blocks or knots from our mind and experiencing unending peace and continuous happiness.

Once our mind is free of all inner obstructions it is like a clear, infinite blue sky, completely peaceful and free from any problems. At the moment our mind is like a cloudy sky, sometimes very stormy, generally gray with only a little occasional clarity.

We can use the second Reiki symbol to gradually release the inner knots within our mind. We start by dealing with the problems, anxieties, or addictions that are most obvious or serious and we work toward revealing and healing our more subtle negative tendencies. Partly it is simply a process of getting to know ourselves, watching our own mind and how we react in certain situations. Training in watching our mind is a great way to inner peace and self-understanding. Once we have become familiar with this practice we can begin to change our behavior patterns but the first stage is simply learning to "watch" or develop self-awareness. After a while we may begin to notice that we are quite an impatient person. Perhaps we get easily irritated when stuck in traffic or we easily say sharp words or criticize. We may begin to notice that we are lonely but that our busy life has previously hidden this feeling. Many people begin to notice a constant lack of mental peace or mild depression; again these feelings might have been hidden by the distractions of a busy life.

Gradually, though, if we continue to train ourselves in developing the opposing positive states of mind these unpleasant states of mind will subside and we will develop a lasting inner peace and clarity of mind. We have to be patient with ourselves and practice training and healing the mind on a daily basis to gain lasting results.

Eventually we will notice that all negative or unpleasant states of mind revolve around a sense of "I" or "Me" as being the most important person in the world. This realization is a great step forward because we are beginning to identify the very root of all unhappiness. Transforming self-concern into concern for the welfare of others is the path to liberation from all problems and unhappiness. Abandoning ourselves or sense of "I" or losing our "self" in cherishing others is a very liberating and enjoyable experience.

So this is our main task, to gradually and steadily eliminate self-obsession and develop a well-balanced and compassionate way of being. This of course does not mean that we have to physically go out and "save the world," it is principally an inner transformation that we are looking for. Also no one has to know what we are doing, an old Tibetan Buddhist saying teaches us to "remain natural whilst changing our aspiration." Also we do not become a "doormat" for others since this might serve only to increase their selfishness by taking advantage of our kindness. So we need to be skillful and develop wisdom alongside compassion. If we have a compassionate nature we can still use strong words and actions when they are needed. If we feel that being passive is not helping or making a situation worse we should speak or act appropriately while still keeping a good motivation.

When to use the second symbol

There are lots of practical situations where we can use the second symbol on a daily basis. Many are similar to those mentioned for the first symbol and again we need to encourage ourselves to be creative and develop a special relationship with the symbol. We cannot hurt ourselves or anybody else with these symbols so we need to develop the confidence to use them as often as possible until we begin to see what situations they are most effective in.

The most obvious way we can use this symbol is during a Reiki session. We would create and activate the symbol over our own palms to begin with. Some practitioners like to do this over the crown, throat, and heart chakras, which can be a powerful healing experience in itself. Then another option, before the healing session begins, is to create and activate a very large second symbol in the center of the room. Some practitioners also like to accompany this with a large power symbol on each wall. We can do all of these things or just simply the palms and heart, whatever feels right to us.

When the healing begins we simply follow the routine for first degree, i.e. the normal twelve positions of Reiki and as mentioned earlier we can reduce the treatment time if we wish as second degree is more powerful. Just before we begin the first position we need to create and activate the second symbol over the crown chakra of the patient. Again, some practitioners like to take this farther and repeat this for the throat and heart chakras but this is optional. Another option is to very gently blow on the symbol we have created over the crown and visualize it moving down through the throat chakra and into the heart area. If we can master this gentle practice it can be quite a special way to begin and end a treatment. But again it can be quite powerful and "shift" or loosen a lot of inner baggage so gently does it.

As with the power symbol, before we create and activate a mental and emotional healing symbol, we need to make an intention. This can simply be "may this symbol work for this person's greatest good" or we can be specific: "may this symbol work to help this person overcome depression or stop smoking, transform their approach to life, be more positive, more understanding, kinder, more tolerant, improve their memory, improve clarity of mind, improve wisdom" and so on.

Setting the intention is important and setting an intention that is closest to what the patient actually needs rather than what we or even they think they need is most important. If our intuition or inner wisdom is good we can use it; if sometimes it is lacking then we need to just hand the situation over to Reiki. Just being a channel is the most simple, easy, and often most rewarding method.

Throughout the treatment we can continue to create and activate more mental and emotional symbols. This might be especially appropriate if we come to a part of the body that we feel is particularly associated with a mental or emotional problem, or if an inner problem is plainly manifesting as an outer one. For example, back strain can be symbolic of carrying too much responsibility and using the second symbol on the strained area can have a direct effect on that part of the mind that needs to change. It could help that kind of person become mentally stronger or help them to share their problems with others or cause them to become more able to delegate and organize their workload. However, although this way of healing can be helpful we can overdo it and become too involved with trying to direct Reiki. So keeping a mental eye on ourselves is really useful!

Also we need to mentally check our motivation for giving Reiki to others from time to time. A purely altruistic motivation takes time to develop but it is a goal well worth working toward. As we progress in our practice and as we begin to get to know ourselves a little better we may not like what we find or what Reiki reveals. Reiki is like a mirror of the soul or mind. The closer our relationship with this special force for good the clearer we see ourselves. This is a wonderful process but obviously challenging. We do it in stages, we do it gradually, and we do it consistently. Sometimes we need to be brave and trusting because it is the trust that opens our mind to the deepest levels of inner healing and the stages to enlightenment or perfection of wisdom. Without trust or faith our mind remains closed tight like a clam and the work we do on ourselves will always be superficial. If we really want what Reiki has to offer we need to make a special effort to open our heart and mind and let the "perfect consciousness" touch and gradually perfect our own.

Some Masters teach a special hand position for mental and emotional healing. If the patient is on their back this involves cradling the back of the head (the occipital) with the palm of one hand, perhaps the left, and placing the other over the crown of the head, with the fingers just touching the top of the forehead.

Other Masters teach that we do not need to deviate from the original twelve positions. It is really a case of personal choice and what seems to work well with individual clients. It is now well known that the way Dr. Usui used Reiki was much more "free-form" than we originally thought in the West.

Obviously we can spend longer on the head and heart areas, which are connected strongly with mental and emotional healing, the brain being the tool through which the mind perceives and communicates with the world and the heart being the location of our actual root or very subtle mind. The heart is also the place we point to when we say things like "What about me?" indicating that our sense of self is generally located here. We cling and dearly protect this sense of "I" in fact all the decisions we make in life are based on satisfying our sense of "I." Yet when our mind is quiet and we try to really look within we have difficulty in finding this "I," it seems to become very illusory and far less obvious the more we try to look for it!

In fact losing our sense of "I" completely or seeing it for what it really is, just a mental projection, is a very freeing experience. Hawayo Takata, a well-known Reiki Master, said "No I.... just like that you will find lasting health and happiness."

As mentioned we can also use the second symbol on a daily basis in a similar way to the power symbol. We can use it on friends and family and other people or situations without them being aware that we are helping. It can be like a silent or secret healing blessing for body and mind. We do not need to touch, we just set our intention and create/activate the symbol as explained in the next section. It might now be worth re-reading the section on the various uses for the power symbol and writing down what kind of situations you personally might be able to use it in and also what circumstances might especially merit using the mental and emotional healing symbol.

Remember that the symbols have a special energy or life force of their own; they are pure Reiki. If we allow them to work through us without too much interference from our side this can be the most effective way of "living" second degree Reiki. Although second degree Reiki gives us tools that we can consciously use to improve our practice and experience we are also being asked to relinquish our grip on what we think is right and wrong or black and white. So although we are given more responsibility we can really only fulfill this role by abandoning our judgment and allowing a greater force for good to bless, guide, and direct us in our life's journey to benefit others and fulfill our potential for great happiness and understanding. If we want to progress along this path quickly it is worth remembering that ordinary minds perceive ordinary environments and ordinary people. A mind that relates to the great potential for happiness and goodness in ourselves and others, and strives to achieve this, lives in an extraordinary world and encounters only heroes and heroines.

The other obvious use of the mental and emotional healing symbol is, as mentioned at the beginning of this section, for our own spiritual development. We can use the symbol as an object of meditation or simply incorporate it into our daily or weekly routine of self-treatment. We can set specific intentions like "I would like to use this symbol to develop greater compassion and patience, overcome my miserliness, develop confidence and inner strength" or something similar. Or again we can hand over our desires to Reiki and ask for what we really need at this point in our spiritual growth. It is possible that Reiki will point you toward other spiritual paths or traditions. Go along with what Reiki is showing you and asking you to look at, it will be worthwhile, truly rewarding, and ultimately enlightening!

Reiki is simply an emanation of the truth or greatest good, just like most other spiritual traditions, so there should be no difficulty walking a genuine spiritual path to enlightenment or communion with God whilst still using Reiki to help yourself and others. Trust your own judgment and listen to your own inner wisdom. We are simply surrendering ourselves to our own potential for good, not to the control of others. However, it might be the case that Reiki leads us to another spiritual tradition that we feel is right for us and then it might happen that Reiki takes on more of a secondary or supporting role for us.

Healing the past and creating the future

One of the most interesting and wonderful aspects of the second Reiki symbol is that we can use it to heal the past and create the future. It seems amazing and perhaps a little far-fetched when we are first given this knowledge. But in time it becomes second nature and the more we get to know Reiki and our own mind the more natural and spontaneous these healing and creative actions will become.

We know the mental and emotional healing symbol is a wonderful tool for healing difficulties that we are facing at present. However, we rarely stop to think that many of the issues we carry at the moment are the fruit of past traumatic incidents that made such a deep impression on our consciousness that the waves or repercussions are still being felt. We know that small "incidents" can have a profound effect on the vulnerable mind of a child and often adults don't notice this or tell the child to simply forget about it. Indeed, the child might forget about it without actually coming to terms with it. In this case it makes it very difficult later in life to clearly identify the cause of some personality disorder or emotional weakness.

Many people spend years in therapy trying to solve and heal such problems, sometimes with successful results. We are very fortunate to have a special opportunity to heal these difficulties easily and without experiencing great trauma. This symbol sends Reiki right to the heart of the matter to bless, heal, and release whatever trauma we might still be carrying within. We do this simply by setting an honest intention, either for specific past trauma or general healing, and being willing to "go with" the healing process however that may manifest. We do not need to worry Reiki will not and cannot harm us. Reiki will never push us beyond our limits so it is completely safe to keep setting these special intentions for deep inner healing for ourselves and others.

In a similar way we can send Reiki to specific future events for ourselves, our family, friends and others, or simply to every future moment of this life and even all our future lives! This makes life a lot more meaningful and enjoyable. However, we have to remember that Reiki brings us what we need and we don't always have the wisdom to understand the value of some of these challenges until sometime later, perhaps even years later. So we need to be patient and make an effort from our own side to make the most of all the challenges and opportunities that life brings us, even the tough ones.

From a Western perspective this might seem like a very strange way of looking at life, especially as we spend so much time trying to avoid all kinds of suffering and even minor annoyances. In fact our whole society and way of life is geared to making the external world an easy and pleasant place to live. Obviously no one wants suffering of any kind; this is a perfectly natural wish but if we look back over our lives generally we can see that the difficulties we have experienced have often led to greater wisdom, understanding, self acceptance, empathy, and compassion. If we had led a charmed life we wouldn't be half the person we are today.

We can see that children who are spoiled and always get their own way often grow up to be selfish, demanding, discontent, and even dangerous adults. So simply by changing our minds we can begin to view difficult situations as opportunities to develop special inner qualities. This attitude shows great wisdom and leads to great peace of mind and future happiness.

The actual process for sending healing to the past and future is explained in the Distant Healing Symbol section.

How to use the second symbol

The mental and emotional healing symbol should always be used in conjunction with the power symbol. If we want to use the symbol for a specific purpose, say to help us develop more patience, confidence, or compassion we simply set our intention, then create and activate the power symbol as previously explained. Then we create and activate the second symbol in the same way and complete the process by once again creating and activating another power symbol. This creates a kind of energetic sandwich with the mental and emotional healing symbol between two power symbols. We can use it daily with the same intention if we want to get long-lasting results and if we have time we can combine it with a self-treatment or meditation. The results we wish for will only come about if we are willing to help Reiki by putting in a little work from our own side and assuming that what we wish for is for our own and others "greatest good." If we get poor results from our intentions and self-treatment we need to reassess our intentions and perhaps start again with more realistic, worthwhile, or honest goals. This is all part of the learning process, which takes time; no one ever achieved enlightenment overnight or without considerable effort. It is not a race but likewise we won't progress without a steady and strong wish to improve ourselves for the good of all.

To create a symbol as previously explained we can simply draw it in the air with our hand or visualize it being drawn or just appearing as light of any appropriate color. To activate it we simply say or think the name three times. Again it is important to mention that these symbols are sacred and special and we should only draw them in the air or say their names when we are alone or in the presence of other advanced Reiki practitioners.

If we want to use this symbol when we are healing others we simply add it to the power symbol at the start of the treatment, as previously explained, and close the "sandwich" with another power symbol. Again we can use it throughout the treatment as with the power symbol. Sometimes it can be a special experience simply to visualize it while we are giving and receiving Reiki. We can use our imagination or just open our mind to whatever way the symbol would like to appear; it might appear surrounded by an aura of light or with a revolving circle of smaller power symbols around it. It may even transform into another symbolic form like a lion, dove, snow-capped mountain, image of Buddha, and so on. We can try to interpret the meanings of such symbols but often it is better just to trust that some special healing is happening on some deep or subtle level and just allow that to continue. Of course if we ever feel overwhelmed by what we are experiencing through using the symbols we can just stop and go for a walk or have a cup of coffee and a biscuit! Exercising our right to take things at our own pace is another useful lesson well learned.

The distant healing symbol

All four of the original Reiki symbols have a special character or energy of their own. With experience of working with them we will get to know them well almost like close friends. The distant healing symbol has many special qualities in its own right although these are often overlooked as it is mainly used to send Reiki "long distance" in terms of space and time.

This symbol has two main meanings or definitions. The name can be translated as "the gateway between Heaven and Earth" and as "this person has proper consciousness."

From the point of view of sending Reiki "long distance" we can see why it is described as a gateway or bridge between the source of Reiki and the person we wish to send Reiki to. The second meaning is not so clear. This is almost like an intention for the recipient's greatest good inclusive within the essence of the symbol. Perhaps this is present so as to keep the gateway or bridge strong and clear and to ensure that whatever we wish for the patient they will only ever receive what they need for their greatest good. This meaning is an indication of the essence and intention of all Reiki. Reiki is simply taking us toward "proper consciousness" which put another way is simply the greatest or purest level of happiness and wisdom.

Because of the special meaning of this symbol meditations on its meaning can be especially powerful for Reiki practitioners. We may think that it is not a symbol for personal healing and that it is only useful for healing others whom we cannot treat directly. But this is not necessarily the case. Because this symbols enables us to work beyond the realms of time and space it has many special uses for us as individual practitioners. For example, we can send Reiki back in time to heal past trauma for ourselves and others and forward in time to make the remaining years of this life a special and meaningful experience. We can work beyond this life and send Reiki to our past lives, which can have a profound effect on the person we are now since all that we are at present is ripening karma resulting from our good and negative actions in previous lives. If we can heal or purify past negative karma this can improve our quality of life immeasurably. The practice of purification is central to the Buddhist way of life.

One of the amazing things about using this symbol is that a full treatment can be sent and received in just fifteen minutes and that the power of the healing is not diminished in any way by distance or time. In fact it is often found that the power of a distant Reiki session is more powerful than a hands on. Why this should be is not clear although it might have something to do with the fact that we are fully handing the situation to Reiki since we cannot be with the patient in person. Perhaps this also creates less personality barriers, which sometimes Reiki has to reduce before a pure level of healing can come through.

Two of the questions new second degree practitioners usually ask are "Can I send Reiki to more than one person at a time?" and "Can I send Reiki to someone without asking them?" Of course the answer is yes on both counts. Some people may have scruples about sending Reiki without being asked but Reiki, like Buddha or God is everywhere all the time, in fact every living being is being helped by Reiki every moment according to what their karma will allow. Also we know that Reiki only ever works for the greatest good of all. So even if we try to use specific intentions with distant Reiki to try to change a person's personality this will only work if it is right for them. We can never use Reiki in a manipulative way even if our intentions are good. If you think someone needs Reiki just send it with an intention for them to receive whatever help they need from Reiki. This is often a good way for Reiki people to share Reiki with their partners or family if they are non-Reiki people. Obviously we do not want to tell others we are going to send them Reiki whether they like it or not! Sometimes we might actually find that when we sit down to send others Reiki we get a strong feeling that now is not the right time to send them Reiki. We may even see a picture of them in our mind's eye saying, "No thanks, I'm not ready for this yet, maybe next year" or something similar. Conversely we may see them nodding and saying "Yes please, this is just what I need now." It is good to trust these intuitions and if we don't have a strong intuition either way we can just send it, as Reiki can never harm.

There is no limit to the number of people or situations we can send Reiki to. In fact many second degree practitioners send Reiki to all living beings every day, simply by using an all-encompassing intention. They might start by identifying certain people they are specifically trying to help and certain issues they are working on in their own life then maybe certain major crises or disasters around the world and then all living beings throughout all realms of existence. This is a wonderful thing to do on a daily basis; we can help so many people and accumulate vast amounts of positive karma. In fact we can replace our usual self-treatment that would last about half an hour with this method, which only takes fifteen minutes.

Another special use for this symbol is to send Reiki to people/animals/beings who have died and are in the "intermediate state" between death and rebirth. When any living being dies the consciousness dissolves or transcends inward in the same way it does when we fall asleep, then at the time of death the connection between the body and mind is broken (unlike during sleep) and the mind leaves the body and enters the intermediate state which is similar to the dream state.

If we are able to be with someone when they are dying this is an ideal time to give them Reiki because the state of mind with which we die is really important. If we die with a peaceful happy mind this is wonderful because we enter the intermediate state in a good frame of mind and this ensures that good karma will ripen and we will take a fortunate rebirth. When someone is approaching the time of death we also need to try to keep a peaceful and happy mind. Of course this might not be easy but if we really care about the person who is about to leave this life we need to be in a frame of mind that will most help them. If we are clinging onto them and crying this will cause them anxiety and they may die holding this negativity in their mind.

As mentioned earlier it can be very helpful to gently touch or stroke the crown of a person who is dying. We can do this occasionally during the last few weeks of life and perhaps more frequently when the time of death approaches, although we shouldn't overdo it so as to cause irritation. This simple loving action encourages the mind to leave the body through the crown, which again helps to create the right conditions for a fortunate rebirth in a special place. We don't need to give Reiki to a dying person in a formal way. Simply holding their hands, talking to them gently, or silently praying for their welfare is enough to create the energetic bridge between Reiki practitioner and recipient.

When the mind leaves the body and enters the intermediate state it may remain there for a few days or a few weeks at the most. We can continue sending someone Reiki during this time; it will help them greatly. We can do this in the same way we would normally send absentee Reiki, as outlined below. If they are entering the human realm again they will take rebirth at the moment of conception, the mind entering the union of the father's sperm and mother's egg. So we can even continue sending them Reiki during the time they spend inside their new mother and on throughout their childhood! There are no limitations with Reiki.

It is of course difficult for us to know where someone is taking rebirth, as there are countless different realms of existence. The best thing we can do is to pray and send them Reiki for their greatest good, wishing them to find lasting happiness and maybe find a spiritual path that will lead them to enlightenment, since this is the greatest happiness anyone could ever have. Of course if we don't feel comfortable with this, or can't accept that we take rebirth, this will not affect the Reiki we send to people after death, it is still a very special Reiki practice.

While we are on the subject, Buddhists believe that the only way to escape the endless cycle of birth, ageing, sickness, death, and rebirth is to attain full enlightenment or our full inner or spiritual potential. Then we are also in a position to help others achieve the same state of pure happiness and complete wisdom, indeed when we become a Buddha this is our sole purpose, just as it is the nature of the sun to give warmth and light. An enlightened being cannot help but benefit others in whatever way is best for them, it is a spontaneous and natural wish, this special intention is the very nature of a Buddha.

How to use the distant healing symbol

Like the other symbols the distant healing symbol is simple to use. When you learn second degree your Reiki teacher will show you the symbol for the first time and tell you its name and how to use it in conjunction with the power symbol and the mental and emotional symbol. All three have to be used together when practicing distant healing.

Usually the first two symbols are taught on the first day of the course and the third symbol is given on the second day. It is the most difficult symbol to draw and memorize. But often because of the special nature of these symbols they are learnt quite easily. Your teacher will probably show you how to break the symbol up into four parts, learn each part then put the whole thing together and within a few days you will be using it easily. If your teacher allows you to write the symbol down and take it home, which was never originally allowed, try to memorize it as soon as possible and destroy the written copy. This is really for your own benefit. The more we can keep Reiki true to its origins the longer it will remain in this world.

The first stage is that we need to bring to mind the person, people, or situation we want to send Reiki to. If it is one or just a few individuals we can simply bring them to mind and say each of their names three times quietly to ourselves. It doesn't matter if we cannot visualize them clearly in our mind: intention is everything. If it is a situation or maybe a natural disaster we see on the news, again we bring that situation to mind and give it an appropriate name and think/say this name three times.

Then we set our intention. Sometimes it is better to think of the intention before we do the first stage then we can go straight into the correct intention without breaking our concentration. If we are in doubt about the correct intention we simply use the tried and tested "for their greatest good."

If we are sending Reiki to one person we need to draw the symbol over the head of the visualized person, so that the bottom part of the symbol ends over the forehead and not going below the eyebrows. If we think about how the distant healing symbol is made up we will see that it can be split up into four parts. Your Master may have already shown you this as a way to help you remember how to draw it. If we find it easier we can draw the symbol over the head of the patient in our imagination, in four parts, each one being overlaid by the next. If we are alone we can physically draw the symbol in the air at the same time, which sometimes helps.

If we want to send Reiki to many people we do not need to draw the symbol for each person. We can imagine all the faces receiving a symbol over their heads at the same time or again, if we find it difficult to visualize clearly, just remember that our intention to send Reiki to these people is enough. Once we have set the process in motion they will receive all that they need. Having confidence in this process helps us to develop a special relationship with Reiki and become a clearer channel. Once we have drawn the distant healing symbol we activate it by quietly saying its name three times. We then draw and activate a power symbol directly over the distant symbol, we follow this with a mental and emotional healing symbol, and then another power symbol to seal and complete the intention to send Reiki. Then the treatment begins.

During the first five minutes the four head positions are treated, then the four front positions during the second five minutes, and the four back positions during the last five minutes. During the fifteen minutes we do not need to mentally think about the people we are sending Reiki to; all we need to do is place both our hands on our right knee to represent the four head positions, then move our hands, without breaking contact with our own body, to our right thigh for the second five minutes. Then finally we move our hands slowly across our body, again without breaking contact with our own body, to our left thigh, which represents the four back positions of a full Reiki treatment.

As with all Reiki healing we do not need to visualize or meditate, just relax and enjoy. But if we wish we can visualize our patients receiving Reiki as white or golden light, we can imagine that all their sickness and worries are completely removed and that they are happy, relaxed, and healthy. Then we can generate a sincere and relaxed mind of joy, just believing, like a child, that this has actually happened, then we focus or concentrate on that mind of belief/joy. Some days it may be helpful to practice this visualization on ourselves, in the same way we just believe that all our worries and problems have been taken away and we are happy, content, and healthy. When we do this meditation for our own benefit it will be even more powerful if we do it with a motivation of wishing to use the benefits we derive to help others. We can set a simple intention at the start like "May this healing meditation be for the greatest benefit of all living beings" or something similar.

We can use other hand positions during an absentee treatment, those mentioned above are helpful if we are seated upright as they allow us to relax the arms, which helps us to keep a relaxed mind and enjoy receiving Reiki ourselves. Incidentally we can always include ourselves in the list of people to send absentee Reiki to. That way we receive a full treatment as well.

If you are lying down, three good positions to choose are one of the head positions, the heart, and the groin position or choose any other three positions that suit you. The reason we use three positions is that Reiki seems to be sent more constantly and strongly than if we just make a mental intention and let Reiki do the rest. We also benefit greatly by being more involved with the process. Also, because we obviously have a strong karmic connection with our Reiki patients maybe Reiki uses this as a channel to reach those who may not yet have developed such a close relationship with Reiki.

It is possible to send an absentee treatment even if we are busy, i.e. at work, whilst driving, shopping, playing with the kids. To do this we do need a couple of minutes to set our intention and set up the treatment by creating and activating the symbols. Then all we need to do is to use the thumb and first finger of one hand to mark the passing of each five-minute period. For the first five minutes we lightly hold the thumb against the first section of the forefinger, then move it to the second section for the duration of the second five minute period and then without breaking contact with the finger move the thumb so that it is touching the third section of the forefinger for the last period of the Reiki treatment.

Amazingly this can work just as well for the recipient as the normal way of sending Reiki. The only downside is that we do not benefit as much as it can be more difficult to appreciate receiving Reiki ourselves when we are physically very active. Although by learning to keep our mind calm even when we are busy it is possible to still receive Reiki blessings. The main barrier to receiving benefit from Reiki is an agitated mind.

When we are sending an absentee treatment as mentioned we

can just switch off, relax, and receive whatever we need as well or we can take a more active role in the healing process by imagining that we are sending symbols to specific physical places in the recipient's body for specific mental and emotional healing purposes. This process is the same as that outlined in the sections on how to use the first and second symbol, the only difference is that we have to imagine that we are actually with the recipient or that we are sending the symbols to the patient or again we can just make our intention for specific healing and Reiki will do the rest.

With time and experience we will develop excellent healing skills that work well and that we have great confidence in.

Some Reiki practitioners like to use photographs to send Reiki to others. If we have a photo we set our intention then simply draw the symbols over the photo. Alternatively we can draw a simple outline of a head and shoulders then write the name of the patient in this and draw the symbols over it. You may come up with other ideas that work well for you.

The reiki crystal method

This combines the absentee technique with crystals to create a constant flow of powerful Reiki to many people, so that the recipients can receive Reiki 24 hours a day for as long as necessary. This technique is explained in Appendix 2.

Sending Reiki to past and future situations

This is one of the amazing characteristics of Reiki. At first, however, it might seem a little far-fetched: are we actually able to go backwards and forwards in time? Can we visit the past and change the way things happened? Can we visit the future and arrange things so that we can know for certain what will happen? These are great questions to contemplate.

We are taught that there are no limits to what we can do or

achieve with Reiki. Maybe we have confidence in Reiki as a healing technique but do not wish to look any deeper into what Reiki really is, its very essence. These questions can make us feel a little uncomfortable because if we wish to know the answers to these questions we need to know who we are, we need to look within our own mind, to get in touch with and discover our own essence. This can be a wonderfully exciting journey to the center of our own reality, discovering the secrets of creation, the ultimate nature of reality. But this may not be everyone's cup of tea! For the time being all we need to know is that we can send Reiki to past and future situations with great results. This is how we do it.

Firstly we bring the situation to mind. If it is very upsetting for us we do not need to dwell on it too long. But if we can it is useful to remember or visualize the situation as clearly as we can for a few minutes, bringing to mind the people, thoughts, and emotions that go with it. Then we can give the situation a rough name like "the day I was born," "my first day at school," "when my Dad died," "last week's argument with a friend," "the interview next week," "my career," "my children's future," etc. There really are no limits to the situations we can send Reiki to. It can be really beneficial to spend some time making a list of all the difficult or traumatic experiences we have been through in this life, then we can send Reiki to each of them, perhaps concentrating on one event each week and doing an absentee treatment each day. Or we can do one a day or simply send Reiki to them all during one session, whatever we feel will be most effective and healing for us. Sometimes healing a past situation at the same time of year it happened can be really effective; we can even go as far as healing that situation at the same date and time. For example, on our birthday we could send Reiki back in time at exactly the time we were born; this can be quite a powerful healing experience and can help us rediscover our purpose or mission in life. Before we begin we can ask ourselves questions like "What is the main purpose of my being born in this world?" or "How can I use the rest of my life to really fulfill my potential?" Other special days might be when you became an adult, your first partner, the day you were married, the day someone close to you died. You could even make a list of these "special" events and spend a year sending healing Reiki to these inner memories, each on the appropriate date. Of course we can do this for other people as well.

If we feel some things are going to take time to heal or work through then we need to adopt a sensible attitude and work steadily toward our own healing. But it can also be useful to remember that the past is only a memory, simply pictures in our mind that can evoke powerful emotions. If we can generate some clear thinking and realize that whatever problems and difficulties we have experienced in the past have passed and are now simply recollections in our own mind, we can let them go and Reiki can help us move on much more swiftly and smoothly.

The next step is to set our intention. That is what we want to do or see happen in the future and what we want to do with the past. Some Reiki teachers say that we can actually change the past, actually visit the past and change what happened. Even if this were possible we would have to be careful about what we did since all our actions affect so many others. If our motivation is not completely pure and we choose to change things without clearly knowing the consequences we can actually be creating more problems and confusion in the "great scheme of things." Generally it is best just to ask Reiki to bless any situation or problems we have previously encountered always "for the greatest good of all."

When dealing with future events, again it is generally better to set our intention "for the greatest good" especially if we are not sure what would be the best intention to set. But for everyday situations like interviews, relationships, money worries, health, etc. we can use whatever kind of intentions we wish and we can always qualify them with "if it is for the greatest good of all." Then we simply continue creating and activating the symbols as we would for a normal absentee treatment. Just bring to mind a rough image of the situation, make your intention, and mentally draw the symbols over this image in your mind. Again, don't worry if you can't see things clearly in your mind; intention is everything. During the treatment you can continue mentally drawing and activating symbols for different people and with different intentions or you can simply relax and let Reiki do what is needed.

Sometimes when we do the latter we get glimpses of what Reiki is doing, people's faces appear in our mind, perhaps with symbols over them, maybe their expression tells a story. We can also get an indication of what Reiki wants us to do with our life, especially if that was our intention or question to Reiki at the start of the treatment. In short we can ask Reiki to heal our past and sort our future out, then sit back watch and wait for directions and good advice, which may come from obvious or unexpected places!

Purifying negative karma

It is wonderful to heal our own traumas in the past but it is also really important to bring to mind the times we have hurt others. In many ways these situations are the ones we really need to concentrate on because sooner or later this karma will come back to us and we need to neutralize or purify it before we experience the unpleasant consequences of our past negative actions. Purifying negative karma is not something that is taught when we learn Reiki. There follows a simple technique that is derived from Buddhist understanding that we can try. But if we want to be sure we are correctly purifying we need to study appropriate books or seek advice from a qualified teacher (see Appendix 4 and 5).

First we need to generate a good motivation, thinking "may all beings benefit from this healing" or "through my healing these traumas (or purifying this negative karma) and relying on Reiki may I eventually attain enlightenment for the benefit of others."

Then we need to mentally generate regret (not guilt) for any negativity we may have created in the past. For example, if there were times when we hurt others or acted selfishly this is a really good opportunity to generate some regret in our mind without being hard on ourselves. Regret is a very positive mind; it is very different from guilt. If we have strong regret and this leads to an inner resolution to abandon selfishness, impatience, anger, etc. this is wonderful. This is a very special and mature process of contemplation and decision. Once we have generated sincere regret and made a promise not to commit similar negative actions in the future, we continue with the absentee treatment process. As part of the purification process we can also think of some positive action that we feel would help to "put things right"; this might be giving more Reiki to people, helping others in some way, doing more meditation, etc.

If we hurt someone else it is also really important that we sincerely wish for them to find lasting happiness and peace of mind. We can send them Reiki with this intention as part of the absentee treatment, then we can imagine the negative karma that we created is completely purified and we are released from having to experience this particular karma. If we wish, during the treatment, we can visualize our own negative karma as a black ball of dense smoke at our heart, which gradually dissolves in the light of Reiki until it completely disappears. Then we try to concentrate on enjoying the feeling of being free and happy that our karma is purified.

The best way to avoid creating negative karma is to always maintain a good heart toward others. Purifying negative karma is one of the most important aspects of the spiritual path, without this it is impossible to progress. Developing a deep experience of compassion purifies negative karma, also from a Buddhist perspective developing our wisdom purifies karma, especially our understanding and experience of "emptiness", the ultimate nature of reality. In Buddhism there are special meditation techniques and methods to swiftly purify negative karma (for more information see *Joyful Path of Good Fortune* by Geshe Kelsang Gyatso, Tharpa Books).

Dedication

As always when we have finished our absentee treatment we need to dedicate our good karma for a positive purpose then it cannot be damaged or dissipated. We can think "Through the force of this virtuous action of sending Reiki may all beings be free from suffering and find lasting peace and happiness." If we want to lead others to a state of lasting happiness we need to achieve it ourselves first so a more appropriate wish might be "Through the force of these virtuous actions may I swiftly attain the supreme wisdom of full enlightenment for the benefit of others."

7

The Master symbol

Where is now?!

We have no choice – life is a journey from birth to death. What we do in between those major events is really important. There is another journey we can take during this time and this is a journey of choice. Maybe many Reiki practitioners do not want to take this journey for the time being. But as second degree practitioners and Reiki teachers we have to acknowledge that with Reiki we are being drawn toward realizing our own true nature, toward directly experiencing the innate clarity and purity of our own consciousness, very subtle mind, or soul. All religions believe there is a benevolent force in the universe, which is pure love and wisdom, and we all try to develop a deep relationship, communion, or union with this supreme consciousness.

On our own we are powerless, vulnerable, and fragile but with God/Buddha/The Great Spirit all things are possible. With this special relationship we can make our precious human life really meaningful. We can overcome all fear, anger, jealousy, attachment, and all negative states of mind. We can gradually perfect all our good qualities and draw closer to becoming a deeply spiritual being, able to guide and help others find freedom from all kinds of problems and gain lasting peace of mind and genuine happiness.

The fourth symbol, often called the Master symbol, is the symbolic representation of this special path or journey toward realizing our true nature. By receiving empowerment with this symbol we are planting a "seed" in our mental continuum that with special care and attention will ripen into the realizations of pure compassion and wisdom. The perfection of these special qualities is the true essence of a human life. Human beings fill their lives with many things: relationships, study, careers, accumulating wealth, hobbies and pastimes, but in the end we have to die and leave all these things behind. The only thing we take with us to our future lives are the inner qualities we have developed. If we have spent our time engaging in meaningless activities we have missed a very special opportunity and not understood our potential. As mentioned earlier it is said in the Buddhist scriptures that all beings are trapped within cyclic existence, taking rebirth after rebirth in many different realms of existence and as every conceivable kind of being. Sometimes we take rebirth as humans, sometimes animals or insects, sometimes Gods or spirits. This cycle is endless and most of the rebirths we take are characterized by problems and suffering. Even a human rebirth, which is one of the most fortunate ones, can be very unpleasant. We know that most of the world's population lives in poverty; it is only a minority who have comfortable lives and have the freedom to discover and practice authentic spiritual paths. Even then our life can be plagued by stress, problems with relationships, career, illness, etc., and there are many distractions and responsibilities that pull us away from developing a simple, meaningful, and spiritual life.

We might think how is it possible for a human being to take rebirth as, say, a dog? When our human life comes to an end our body becomes lifeless and our mind leaves our body. Our mind is blown by the winds or energy of our karma. If through previous negative actions we have created the karma or causes to take rebirth as a dog this can easily happen. As mentioned earlier the process of death, intermediate state, and rebirth is very similar to the process of falling asleep, dreaming, and waking up. When we take rebirth it is simply like waking up as a completely different being in a completely different body and we generally have no recollection of our previous body or personality. If we run out of karma to continue being born as a human it is impossible to take a human rebirth. It is simply a matter of cause and effect, albeit a shocking one.

It may be difficult for us to accept these truths at first but if we spend some time looking at the world and the beings around us we will begin to see that the law of karma explains everything and that all beings are inextricably caught up in it. We are very fortunate to have gained a human rebirth – it is very rare. Although there appear to be billions of human beings on this planet, compared to the countless number of beings in the "lower" realms of existence (just think of the number of insects in one garden in summer, above and below ground), a human rebirth is extremely rare. It is even rarer to be a human being and have an interest in the spiritual path, and it is the most rare of rebirths to actually find a clear and authentic spiritual path that leads to full enlightenment. Many of us have the karma to enter and complete this special journey but from our own side we need to realize the value and rarity of this opportunity or we will miss it or only take a half-hearted interest.

In the Buddhist scriptures a human life is compared to a boat: we are able to use this life to cross the river of cyclic suffering and reach the shore of enlightenment within one lifetime. From a Buddhist perspective when we have purified all our negative karma and realized all the stages of the path to enlightenment we will never have to take another uncontrolled rebirth. At the moment we do not know where we shall be reborn in our next life or in what form; we will be blown by the winds of whatever karma is ripening for us at the time of our death.

In the short term we need some immediate protection because of our precarious position and in the medium to long term we need to make a consistent effort to build within our minds the realizations that will remove any possibility of unfortunate rebirth or any kind of suffering.

To prevent lower rebirth we need to firstly create the causes for higher rebirth and remove the causes of lower rebirth. According to the laws of cause and effect or karma the direct cause of a human rebirth is the practice of moral discipline. Moral discipline simply means refraining from negative actions that we feel drawn to commit. In Buddhism there are ten main "non-virtuous" or negative actions and these are separated into three bodily or physical actions (killing, stealing, and sexual misconduct), four verbal actions (lying, divisive speech, hurtful speech, and idle chatter), and three mental actions or attitudes (covetousness, malice, and holding wrong views).

Most of these are self-explanatory. However, good sexual conduct mainly means being faithful to your partner. Holding wrong views means denying the existence of past and future lives, the law of karma, etc. (A full explanation is given in Joyful Path of Good Fortune by Geshe Kelsang Gyatso, Tharpa Publications.)

If we do not feel drawn to commit a negative action then simply not doing it is not a practice of moral discipline. For example, a baby cannot kill or steal but this is not a practice of moral discipline. So to be practicing moral discipline we always need to be looking to improve our behavior or state of mind. It is the actions of controlling or improving our actions or mind that creates the good karma of moral discipline.

We have to be honest with ourselves and look at our life and see where we need to improve and try to make commitments to improve our way of life. Spotting our weaknesses and trying to steadily improve or strengthen them is a very heroic way of life. Nowadays it is very easy to give in and be like others and do whatever we feel like regardless of the consequences and without regard for others. In the face of a society that celebrates promiscuity and selfishness it takes a strong soul to swim against the current. But even if just a few people really try this will have a special effect on the rest of the world and eventually the tide will turn.

We can practice moral discipline simply by abandoning selfish thoughts and actions and trying to cultivate actions of body, speech, and mind that are well intentioned, do not harm others, and where possible benefit others. Everything starts in the mind, all our actions of body and speech come from a thought or emotion so if we try to maintain a good heart all the time (especially when we don't feel like it!) we can be sure that we are practicing moral discipline.

At first we may feel false in our intentions but if we persevere eventually this special way of living will become more natural and spontaneous; with steady effort it is only a matter of time. We do not want to become pious and we need to be careful that we do not develop pride, thinking that others are selfish or ignorant. This would defeat the purpose as we are doing this essentially for the benefit of others. Try to feel that others are more important than yourself and do not try to convert others to your views; just share your wisdom if others are genuinely interested. If they see that your quality of life is good and that you are generally happy and relaxed then one day they will seek your advice.

Also at the time of death we need to make sure that we die with a peaceful mind and feel close to God or Buddha or our own "Higher Nature." Having a peaceful mind at the time of death ensures that good karma will ripen and naturally direct our soul or very subtle mind to a peaceful and beautiful place of rebirth. Just accepting death with a peaceful and happy mind, letting go of any regrets and wishing to use our next life to benefit others is the best type of mind to die with. It is worth taking this advice to heart right now and sharing it with others as the time of our death is uncertain – we may die today. Being ready for death, even if we are young and healthy, is a wise way of life.

In the face of death our life takes on much more meaning. "Death awareness" concentrates the mind and brings us to our senses, it makes us see clearly what is important in life and helps us not to get too caught up in the meaningless pursuit of worldly gain. When we realize that we are mortal, that our life is fragile and our death may be imminent we are forced to take stock and reassess our priorities. Materialistic and selfish attitudes melt away and we become acutely aware of the value of life, all life. If we accept that taking a lower rebirth is possible we also become aware that making the most of our human potential is really important. As humans we have the potential to achieve a state of spiritual development that prevents any kind of lower rebirth in the future. Of all the realms of existence where we can take rebirth the human realm is one of the very few places where we can attain the state of full enlightenment, in just one lifetime. So without hesitation we need to grasp this opportunity.

On the Buddhist path there are three main qualities we need to perfect: renunciation, compassion, and wisdom. Renunciation is the wish to enter, progress along, and complete the spiritual path. This wish is based on the deep understanding that lasting happiness cannot be found in any other way. Compassion is the wish for others to be free from suffering and find everlasting happiness. There are many levels of wisdom, just understanding that happiness is a state of mind and to develop lasting happiness we need to look within, this is wisdom. Wisdom realizing "emptiness" is the most profound level of wisdom. This realization or special level of consciousness frees us from the dream-like prison of cyclic existence. Reiki can help us to develop these qualities to perfection but we need to study authentic spiritual instructions and receive correct teachings to be able to progress successfully.

It is impossible to describe the special attributes of a mind that has perfected these qualities; it is beyond ordinary conception. Such a mind works unceasingly for the benefit of others and, seeing spontaneously and simultaneously all past lives, present, and future potential of all living beings, knows how to help others in the best way possible.

We can say that Reiki is an emanation of this level of perfect and pure loving universal consciousness, which is also our own greatest potential. If we use Reiki with a good motivation it will help us toward our own enlightenment day by day, month by month, year by year. If we take our time and are open to Reiki we can expect excellent results. The most important thing is to create a good motivation in our mind every day. We need to think of others in all we do. The more we familiarize ourselves with the wish to attain enlightenment, so that we can help others, the quicker that will come about. It is impossible to attain enlightenment for our own benefit since such a mind has no sense of selfishness; its only concern is the welfare of others. All spiritual realizations naturally arise in dependence upon reducing self-cherishing or self-importance and perfecting our wish to cherish others.

Obviously this is a big task to complete. So we need to be realistic and take it on as a long-term way of life. Try to think "OK, it may take me a long time to develop these special qualities and there may be times when my old habits get the better of me. But this is something that is really important to me, this is how I want to live, this is the best thing I could do with my life, so I am just going to keep trying and not worry if things get difficult sometimes."

The master symbol

Once you have received the attunement your Reiki Master will show you the Master symbol and tell you its name. This is the culmination of your Reiki training on one level and can be a very special moment. There are no levels higher than Reiki Master so in one sense you have completed your training. In the past it took years to become a Master but nowadays some people say they are a Reiki Master after only a few weekends of training. Because of familiarity from previous lives it is very possible that some of these people are or will become excellent Masters. However, we have to be careful and honest and try to gauge where we really are in our spiritual training. Most of us are really just beginners and that is a great place to be. If we always regard ourselves as beginners we will always be open to learning and expanding our knowledge and experience further. In fact the further we continue along the path of "becoming" a Master the more we realize we know very little, the humbler we feel, and the closer to enlightenment we become. It is the letting go of "I" and becoming completely focused on the welfare of others that is the essence of the path to enlightenment.

The meaning of the master symbol

The translation of the Master symbol name or mantra is "Great Being of the Universe, shine on me, be my friend." We have to remember that this was translated from the Japanese definition that Dr. Usui passed on to his students. He probably explained it using many different phrases. One commonly used by modern Reiki masters is "Store House of the Great Beaming Light," which has a powerful feeling to it.

Being the highest Reiki symbol we can say that it must represent the highest or purest state of being that anyone can attain. We might say that it represents the synthesis or perfection of all good qualities like wisdom and compassion. Its main function is to guide us in our spiritual journey toward the perfection of our own good qualities. The energy it conveys helps us reduce our negative qualities and misunderstanding and develop the inner strength and wish to travel and complete the spiritual path to enlightenment.

When to use the master symbol

We know that Dr. Usui greatly valued this symbol. He didn't teach many Masters so not many people would have known about this symbol; he felt it was very sacred and powerful and needed to be respected and not used carelessly. It is a very powerful symbol; it is like our direct connection with Buddha or God or our own future enlightenment. It is like the Holy Grail or some other sacred object. If we have a special regard for it, this symbol will function in a very special way for us. So it is often taught that we should use it sparingly and for only two purposes: our own and others' greatest good. It should not be used like the first Reiki symbol, which we can use at any time and for any purpose. Some Reiki Masters say that it can be used on a daily basis but we have to be careful that we do not become careless or take it for granted. Some Masters recommend that their students only use it occasionally and only when they know it is appropriate, i.e. when the other Reiki symbols are not up to the job in hand or when something special is called for or when Reiki prompts us to use it. Such a situation might be when we meet someone whom we feel is at a major crossroads in their life and possibly on the verge of a spiritual awakening, or someone whom we feel is on the verge of a downward spiral either physically, mentally, or spiritually. Of course this symbol is appropriate when someone is near death, in the intermediate state (between death and rebirth), or near rebirth. Also we can use it at a time of local, national, and international crisis. Events such as war, famine, major crime, large scale accidents, and so on are very appropriate opportunities for using this symbol. These are all situations that would respond well to the other three symbols and we should generally use these first and only use the Master symbol if we know or if it just feels like it wants to be used. Generally it is helpful to think twice before using the Master symbol. It is very powerful and we have a duty to use this power wisely. If you never experience a time when it feels appropriate to use the Master symbol this is fine.

Because it is such a sublime, profound, and powerful symbol we almost always need to make our intention for the "greatest or highest good." Making specific intentions is generally not recommended unless again we know in our hearts that this is required in a particular situation. Maybe at some point Reiki will put us in a situation where we have to do this to help us learn a particular lesson. The symbol will only ever work for the greatest good so it is better generally not to confuse the situation by becoming too "involved." The more we can let go and allow Reiki to "use" us the closer we will come to our Reiki nature. Once we have received the empowerment and we have made the connection to this symbol, it is within our system and will work to bring us steadily toward our own greatest good. To encourage this process we can meditate on this symbol as part of our own spiritual practice. Again, some Masters say we can do this daily and some suggest only doing this occasionally. We have to be careful that we do not become too "familiar" with the symbol in that we lose our special view of it, but of course we do need to feel close to it. With practice we will learn how to get the balance right.

Also we do not want to go to another extreme, feeling that the symbol is distant from us because it should not be used regularly, or that it is all powerful and should be worshiped; this is obviously not a healthy attitude. We need to feel close to the symbol or the source of the symbol, like a close friendship.

An alternative view

Some Masters nowadays recommend a much more liberal use of the Master symbol. Perhaps this is appropriate for our time. We have to decide for ourselves which feels "right," the best time to do this is during and just after our Reiki Master initiation course as that is the time when our view of how we are going to live as a Reiki Master is clearest. It can be really helpful to spend some time making notes on how you feel about the course, what you experienced, any strong feelings you had about how to live as a Master, and so on. Then we can always refer back to our notes to help to remind us of our good intentions.

One of the greatest obstacles to spiritual realizations is pride. If we feel that we are someone important, that we possess knowledge or power that others do not, that others look up to us, or that we are more advanced or living on a higher plain then this is a big problem. Buddha said that pride is one of the most difficult delusions or negative states of mind to overcome. It is even more dangerous than an angry mind, through receiving blessings and teachings on the practice of patience even very selfish and angry people can change for the better. However, if we are proud it is difficult for us to take any good advice to heart. If we feel that we are always right it is almost impossible for us to learn from others. If we feel that we have attained some level of spiritual attainment and take pride in this then it is impossible for us to move up to a higher level, in fact pride quickly destroys any spiritual attainments that we have. The opposite is also true, if we are humble and try always to feel like a "beginner" and have a mind that is open to learning from others, even if they have no obvious spiritual qualities, then everyone is our spiritual guide and every day is an opportunity to receive blessings and teachings.

Pride is also a very subtle mind, so we have to be vigilant and honest and even ask others to be honest with us and help us by letting us know when we are inflating our own sense of self. We can of course feel special and loved and happy, confident, and fortunate without feeling pride! We can congratulate and encourage ourselves without feeling pride. Also being humble doesn't mean we have to be quiet or shy; there are plenty of outgoing and gregarious people who have a truly humble nature.

Pride just gets in the way and holds us back; it is a poisonous mind and as Reiki practitioners and especially Masters we have to be extra careful as it can creep up on us steadily over months or years. The best way to overcome pride is to always regard others as special and to genuinely feel that we are in their service. Always work for the benefit of others, never thinking about your own gain or good qualities. Always feel like a servant and you will become a true Master.

How to use the master symbol

As mentioned, your teacher/Master will give you the symbol with its name or mantra, which you need to memorize. Nowadays there are some differences in the symbols that some Masters give their students. These differences are only slight and really make no difference to the effectiveness of the symbol. In fact we might be given one symbol by our Master, then another Master might share their symbol with us and we might feel more at home with that symbol. If this is the case we can simply re-attune ourselves using the new symbol or another Master can do this for us. We may feel uncomfortable about showing anyone our symbol and this is a good attitude, unless we are sure about another Master's Reiki lineage it is better not to show them our symbol. It is sacred and special and probably your Master will have asked you not to show anyone else. If we break this promise without a very good reason this will dissipate the power of our Reiki practice. But not to worry if this has happened already, we can apologize to Reiki, send Reiki back in time to the incident and make a fresh promise to respect and use the symbols wisely to the best of our ability.

We draw and activate the Master symbol in the same way as the other symbols; there is no special method. We set our intention, draw the symbol, and activate it by mentally repeating its name three times. Again we need to carefully think about our intention before we set it. If we feel it is appropriate to set a specific intention we can do so, although with such a powerful symbol and especially at the beginning of our Mastership it might be safer to use the "greatest good" especially if we are using the symbol on others. Although something like "healthy body, healthy mind, meaningful life" for ourselves is great, if we are prepared to accept the truth of this in our life!

Unlike the second and third symbol the Master symbol does not need to be empowered with the first Reiki symbol. It stands alone in this respect. In fact we can say that the other Reiki symbols are an aspect or emanation of the Master symbol, this symbol, or what it represents, being the source of all happiness and healing. However, some Masters do teach their students to empower the Master symbol by using the first Reiki symbol before and after the Master symbol. We can try this and see if it makes sense or feels harmonious or not to us. Normally if we are going to use the Master symbol with the other symbols we would begin by setting our intention, using any of the first three symbols as previously described then pause, set a fresh intention for the greatest good, and then draw and activate the Master symbol.

Learning to attune others

One of the most important things your Master will share with you is how to teach Reiki. That is how to attune or empower others, how to create new Reiki practitioners. This is really special and we are very fortunate to be in a position to receive this sacred and beautiful technique of opening others' bodies and minds to the beneficial influence of Reiki. We do not have to possess great spiritual attainments to successfully attune others and the process of attunement is relatively simple. Although at first there will seem like a lot to remember, within a few days or weeks it will become easier and with the blessings of Reiki eventually it will become second nature.

Originally Reiki Masters in the West would train under another Master for a few years, then at the end of the training period if the Master thought they were ready they would be attuned and told how to attune others. Nowadays, like the other Reiki levels, it can be taught over one weekend. This may sound ridiculous and no doubt many people are becoming Masters without having deep understanding or appreciation of what they have received which consequently they will pass on to their students. However, there is no doubt that many people have Reiki imprints from previous lives and are ready to become Masters again as soon as possible. This is wonderful because the more people that can carry the Master level of Reiki energy the better it will be for the whole world, even if that level of energy is a little restricted by the practitioners' lack of appreciation or understanding, which should improve overtime. So, overall, "quick" mastery might just be what the world really needs right now. Times are changing fast, it would only take a few angry minds to destroy the whole world, so we need the good influence of Reiki practitioners and Masters everywhere to help us through this transitional period.

Using the Master symbol is quite simple, which is excellent because we can receive great benefit and help many people without having to possess or develop a deep understanding or awareness of its true nature and meaning. However, if we can try to develop a little of this understanding it will greatly accelerate our spiritual progress and therefore our ability to benefit others.

The essence of the path

Everyone wants to be happy, no one wants to suffer. Happiness is just a state of mind. If we realize the true nature of our mind or consciousness we can release our true potential for sublime unending happiness. It is only by traveling along this path and reaching its conclusion, full enlightenment, that we will fulfill all our wishes for lasting happiness. We will then be in a position to lead others to the same supreme state of happiness and knowledge. All we need to do is to perfect our good qualities and let go of our bad ones. So it is an inner journey that leads to true happiness; we cannot find what we really want in the external world. Buddha explained that experiencing worldly pleasures is like drinking seawater when we are thirsty. It actually increases our thirst. Once we have satisfied our desires, this temporary state of "happiness" or pleasure soon wears off and once again we are searching for someone or something to bring back those happy feelings. In time it just gets worse, in fact we are not unlike junkies always searching for our next shot of happiness. There is rarely any peace or happiness naturally rising from within.

So we have a problem! Recognizing this is a good place to start. Temporarily we can solve our problems in this life by developing special minds such as patience, contentment, compassion, etc.

through meditation/Reiki, and these will bring us great inner peace. But, as mentioned previously, ultimately we need freedom from Samsara, the endless cycle of birth, ageing, sickness and death, because even if we achieve some level of inner peace in this life we cannot be sure that we will continue our inner training in future lives. It is very easy to be distracted from the path and if we take a "lower" rebirth it is impossible to develop spiritual attainments. So we need to travel as far as we can along the path to liberation and enlightenment in this life. Then when we die if we have not completed our training we simply need to wish and pray to continue our training in our next life and this special intention will guide us safely toward such an opportunity.

Liberation and enlightenment is definitely possible, we just need a clear understanding of the true nature of cyclic existence, a wish to leave, either for our own or others' benefit, and then find a sure way out.

This may be controversial, but, from a Reiki perspective, we do not know that we have a clear path to enlightenment. Dr. Usui mainly taught Reiki as a healing technique and a spiritual path but we do not know how far along the path Reiki can take us. There is no doubt that Reiki brings out the best in us up to a point. However, enlightenment will never arise in our mind naturally; we have to know what it is and how to get there intellectually before we can realize it directly.

We have a choice: we can use Reiki as a tool for healing and developing higher states of consciousness or we can use it for healing and helping us along the path to full enlightenment. Then we will be in a position to protect, heal, and guide countless living beings along the same path. If we are interested in this path we need to seek the advice and guidance of a qualified spiritual guide. In the Buddhist tradition this means someone who practices moral discipline, concentration, and wisdom, has sincere love, and compassion for his or her students and has a direct experience of "emptiness." As you can imagine these qualities are quite rare nowadays so we have to check out potential spiritual guides or teachers very carefully.

How does all this relate to the Master symbol? Good question! Well the Master symbol relates to the ultimate or highest level of consciousness or wisdom and it can help us establish this within our own mind. However, we need clear instructions on how to do this, it will not arise naturally without any effort from our side. Without these instructions we might be able to achieve high levels of concentration and experience great inner peace but this will not last forever; sooner or later our karma for experiencing this will run out. We need to develop the special type of wisdom realizing "emptiness," this is the only way to realize our full potential and puts us in a position to be of real lasting benefit to others. This special wisdom, understanding the way things exist or the ultimate nature of phenomena, is the door to liberation.

Liberation or Nirvana is a wonderful state of existence – very pure, very blissful, very peaceful, a stable and unending happiness, which we will never find in cyclic existence. However, there is an even greater state of existence or consciousness than liberation and this is full enlightenment. Comparing liberation to full enlightenment is said to be like comparing the light of a candle flame to the light of the sun! We cannot imagine the power of such a mind: it is boundless, the nature of pure and spontaneous wisdom and compassion.

As mentioned, to enter the path to liberation we first need to understand the faults of cyclic existence, mainly that no one has or ever will find lasting happiness here. Understanding this deeply we try to generate a strong wish to escape either for our own or others' benefit. Then we need to learn the methods for leaving this limited state of existence.

Basically all our problems arise because our mind is pervaded by a lack of wisdom, we have no control or understanding of how or why things happen or exist, we are victims of our own ignorance. We need to gradually erase or clean this ignorance from our mind by developing and perfecting our wisdom and as we do so we will naturally move closer to nirvana, permanent inner peace.

To realize emptiness directly we need a special type of concentration called "tranquil abiding", again we need correct instructions and a qualified guide to achieve this. The development of pure concentration depends upon the practice of pure moral discipline and since most of us do not understand what moral discipline is, again we need correct instructions and a qualified teacher or guide! None of this will arise naturally in the mind. Our mind is a non-physical phenomenon, there was never a time when it did not exist and there never will be. Our mind or Consciousness is timeless, it goes from life to life, body to body without end, unless we attain liberation. We have had countless previous lives, yet liberation has not happened naturally, so we need to grasp this precious opportunity right now. Dr. Usui did not say that liberation would arise naturally through Reiki practice. Reiki will definitely take us in that general direction by bringing out our good qualities, but in itself it may not be enough to liberate us from cyclic existence.

So now we can look again at "emptiness," the ultimate nature of reality, understanding that without training in correct moral discipline and concentration we will never realize it directly. The first helpful thing to understand is that cyclic existence is just a state of mind or an appearance to mind and that a realization of emptiness and liberation itself is also just a state of mind or an appearance to mind.

At the moment the world we inhabit, all the people and places appear to exist outside of and separately from our mind, without depending upon it in any way. But this deceptive appearance is false and misleading and causes us to create all kinds of positive and negative karma that keeps us tightly locked into cyclic existence. It is true that if we accumulate masses of good karma by being a very positive and caring person this can help us to leave cyclic existence but without developing the wisdom realizing emptiness this karma will ripen as temporary high states of existence that will eventually come to an end and then we will take lower rebirth once again. In Buddhism there are instructions for developing masses of positive energy or good karma very quickly. One of these is the practice of the Six Perfections, the main state of mind we need to perfect is wisdom which we are looking at now and the five "supporting" minds are moral discipline, concentration, giving, patience, and effort. (For more information see *Meaningful to Behold* by Geshe Kelsang Gyatso, Tharpa Publications.)

To understand the type of consciousness or wisdom that the fourth Reiki symbol relates to it might be helpful first to look at the concept of time. Where is the past and where is the future? If we look around and try to find the past we cannot find it. The past is just a memory, pictures in the mind. Even the past of just a few moments ago, when you started reading this sentence, is now just a memory. We cannot bring it back in to "real" existence. Where is the future? It only exists as a possibility, a thought or idea of how it might be. This applies even to the very next moment of our reality or existence. If we look for the future we cannot find it anywhere. The past and future only exist within the mind. We cannot find them outside of the mind, this would of course be impossible.

So we might think that the present truly exists; we can be sure of this can't we?! If the present truly exists outside or independently of our own mind then upon close analysis or investigation we should be able to find or identify it clearly. So where is the present? We might say that the moment of existence we are experiencing now is the present. But how long is a moment? It is impossible to find "the" moment of present existence because within one moment there are smaller moments of time and within those moments smaller moments, and so on and so on. Some people say that nothing exists for more than a moment but it would be more accurate to say that nothing truly exists at all. The present exists in the same way as the past and future, just as a mere appearance to our consciousness or mind, like an illusion or mirage that we believe "truly" exists. Our main problem is that we take this mere appearance to be truly existent then we react to all the illusions or appearances that we perceive on a daily basis as "real." Then when things go our way we become very happy and when they don't we become depressed; there is no real inner peace in our minds because of this mistaken view of reality.

Perhaps the easiest way to understand emptiness is to contemplate the dream analogy. In a dream things appear to be truly existent: during sleep our dream world appears as real as our waking world. We can dream about different people, places, relationships, jobs, travel, and so on and in our dreams all these events, people, and places can appear as real as "real life"! But when we wake up we realize that the things we were taking so seriously in our dream were simply a manifestation of our mind, they didn't really exist they just appeared for a while! So it is that in reality "real life" is simply an appearance to mind in the same way as "dream life."

When thinking about emptiness it is important that we do not think that nothing exists and nothing matters – this is not emptiness. Perhaps we can say that "things do exist, but only just" or that there is "almost nothing." Again, as in a dream things seem real but this reality is false. These phrases are very helpful because they capture the truth or inner experience of emptiness and can help reveal it to us in our own mind, rather than it just being intellectual knowledge.

Correct instructions and explanations of emptiness are essential; they help us to develop our wisdom gradually and joyfully. Emptiness cannot be understood overnight, it might take us a few years before we begin to get a feel for it, but if we have good instruction and the support of qualified teachers we can experience wonderful results that really transform our life for the better. (See *Heart of Wisdom* by Geshe Kelsang Gyatso, Tharpa Publications.) The Reiki Master symbol can bring us closer to an understanding of ultimate truth but to gain a direct inner experience of emptiness we need to study special instructions and receive teachings and blessings directly from those who already abide in emptiness.

This special understanding of things as simply an appearance or manifestation of our own mind is a huge concept for us to grasp. It is not necessarily complicated but because we are used to relating to the world around us as separate from our mind and "truly existent" or "real" when someone finally tells us the truth it can seem completely implausible.

Relating to our world as truly existent and separate from our mind causes us lots of problems: we feel great attachment to some objects that appear to our mind, like our family, our car, places we like, etc. We also feel dislike toward some objects like irritating people, dirty places, some types of food, etc. We are driven by these two main minds of attachment and aversion. Always trying to get what we want and avoid what we don't want. Always looking for happiness and trying to avoid suffering by rearranging our external world. We don't understand that all these objects have the same nature or "taste," they arise out of emptiness, and exist just as a projection of our own mind as in a dream, they are simply our own karma (created by our actions in previous lives) appearing to our own mind.

By understanding and experiencing emptiness we gain extraordinary peace of mind and contentment by experiencing freedom from grasping or believing that we and others and our environment exist. Buddha said "everything depends upon the mind." To gain enlightenment all we have to do is know, realize, or simply understand our own mind.

Let's look at karma and emptiness again; the more we think about these subjects the closer we will come to a deeper understanding. All the problems we experience in everyday life are simply negative karma ripening, the results or effects of previous negative or selfishly motivated actions in previous lives. All our positive and negative actions are like seeds within the root mind and when they ripen we experience their effects.

The world around us, all the people, objects, and environments, appear to be external and separate from our mind. It seems to us that our mind is located within our body and exists separately from everyone and everything else. In reality it is much closer to the truth to say that our mind, specifically our root mind, is the creator of all we perceive and experience. When some karmic seeds ripen, for example, we win some money or someone gives us a really nice present, we feel surprised and pleased. We think that we had nothing to do with this nice windfall and that it has come completely out of the blue. It seems that we, or our mind, and the nice thing that has happened to us are very separate and unconnected.

These two things, the mind perceiving the nice surprise and the nice surprise itself, both actually come from the same place. Within us! From deep within our root mind. Again dreams are a wonderful analogy for understanding this amazing phenomenon. If someone were to give us something nice in a dream whilst we were in the dream we would also think that it was a nice surprise and that it was nothing to do with us. However, when we awoke we would realize that our mind had created the whole situation.

As explained earlier the everyday waking world is also a projection of our root mind. As in a dream our environment, our friends, our family, even our own body and sense of self, are all a projection of our root mind. Moment by moment our reality is being thrown up from deep within our own consciousness like waves breaking on the surface of a vast and deep ocean. We can also say that this is our karma ripening moment by moment. At present we are experiencing the karma of being human; when this karma has been exhausted or used up we will experience the karma of dying and taking rebirth. If we have not created the karma to take rebirth as a human we will take rebirth as an animal or some other type of being. The root mind of all living beings has the same qualities; we just appear in different forms on the surface of life according to whatever karma is ripening for us.

Taking a 'higher' rebirth is vital if we want to continue on the spiritual path. Animals have no opportunity to develop spiritual realizations as they do not have the mental faculties and of all the variety of beings we can take rebirth as not many possess the special attributes conducive to attaining full enlightenment. The main cause of taking a human rebirth is the practice of moral discipline or refraining from negative actions and trying to cultivate positive states of mind. Regular and sincere prayer is also a helping factor and also we need to keep a peaceful mind at the time of death, as this will help good karma to ripen. If we can we should pray at the time of death for a rebirth were we can continue our spiritual development, especially with the motivation of doing this in order to benefit others. This selfless motivation is a wonderful intention to have at the time of death.

Earlier we looked at what moral discipline means. All religions have a code of ethics and generally they are very similar, such as not to harm others, not to lie or steal, to be honest and good, to be faithful and pray or meditate daily and so on. Christians have the Ten Commandments, and Buddhists try to avoid the ten non-virtuous actions. One of the simplest and most powerful ways to keep good moral discipline is to always have a good heart toward others.

There is no point in doing advanced spiritual practices if we have no moral discipline; moral discipline is the foundation of all spiritual attainments. When we have some control in our mind we have freedom. We are no longer a slave to our desires and attachments, we have more peace and space in the mind and this naturally leads us to better concentration, which helps us to improve our wisdom.

It is the wisdom understanding the true nature of things, that will finally bring us what we are all looking for, lasting happiness and freedom from suffering.

To summarize, as Reiki teachers and advanced practitioners we have a responsibility to live our lives well and to set a good example. This does not mean pretending to be perfect but simply trying to steadily improve our inner qualities, perhaps with a motivation to benefit all for the greatest good.

8

A NEW SYMBOL

The greatest good

If we have read the preceding pages we should have a good idea that the spiritual path is a very practical and reliable method to solve our daily problems and find lasting happiness and if we understand it well we can share this special inner experience with others.

It is helpful to bear this in mind when we are using or creating new symbols. The four Reiki symbols are pure because their purpose is to increase inner peace of mind and happiness. So when we are looking to create new symbols it is really helpful to keep a pure intention. We don't want to waste time creating symbols to attract money, promotion, fame, etc.

We can intentionally create symbols simply by playing with a pen and paper while thinking about a particular problem or wish. When we think or create a symbol that "captures" either the problem or the solution we can stop. Then we can activate that symbol by drawing it in the air between two power symbols. If it is a symbol that represents a problem we set an intention to solve it or find a solution. If the symbol represents a solution we set an intention for the solution to live. As always we can qualify our intentions with "for the greatest good."

We may discover symbols in our dreams, or they may simply pop into our mind whilst we are daydreaming, arising from the subconscious mind. It may be obvious to us what they mean and how we should use them or this might take time to reveal. Often it is best not to over-analyze, as symbols can work in very subtle and powerful ways simply by our seeing them.

In this chapter I would like to introduce the main "non-Reiki" symbol that I use.

After learning second degree Reiki I became fascinated by symbols and I read books and spoke to lots of people about how they used symbols. I tried using many symbols, some of which seemed to have a very positive effect and some of which seemed of little use. Generally though I found myself always returning to the four main Reiki symbols. It seemed to me that they were far more powerful and useful. So for a couple of years I lost my interest in other symbols completely until I felt ready to become a Reiki teacher. During my first Reiki exchange after becoming a Reiki teacher I was surprised to see a symbol very clearly in my mind's eye.

At the time I was giving Reiki to another person and reciting the mantra of Medicine Buddha, who is the embodiment of the healing power of all the Buddhas. Also the symbol appeared in blue, which is the color of Medicine Buddha. I immediately felt very close to the symbol and felt it had a good energy and deep meaning.

Over the following days and weeks I spent time thinking about it, drawing it, and generally getting to know it. The main feeling I had was that this symbol was a representation of the "greatest good," so that was what I decided to call it. Whenever I used it I would "draw" it, say its name three times, and, like other symbols, create it between two power symbols.

Here is a brief explanation of what the symbol means to me, maybe it will mean different things to you. The first thing that struck me about this symbol was its similarity to a Stupa. A Stupa is a circular tower, which represents the mind of enlightenment. To Buddhists a Stupa is a very sacred object, just seeing or walking around one creates the cause for us to attain enlightenment in the future. A Stupa is usually made up of circular rings (stone, metal,

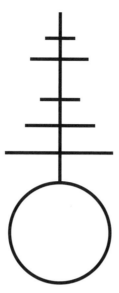

'The Greatest Good'

or wood), which become smaller as the Stupa gains height. Each ring or level represents another stage or realization on the path to enlightenment. The symbol for the greatest good has five levels. This can easily be related to the stages of the path to enlightenment. Also the five levels are split in to two groups.

The first group of three levels can be related to the development of three special spiritual qualities – renunciation, compassion, and wisdom on the path of Sutra. The next two levels can be related to the path of Tantra and represent the spiritual attainments of bliss and emptiness. To attain enlightenment we need to practice and integrate both the paths of Sutra and Tantra.

We have already looked at the importance of developing the three aspects of Sutra and to understand the Tantric path we need to receive teachings from a qualified Tantric teacher. There are not many pure Tantric teachers in this world and the teachings and meditations, although not difficult, are quite profound and need to be combined skillfully with a good understanding of Sutra, which acts as a firm foundation. With this in mind and because not many people will practice Tantra you might feel more comfortable reducing the height of the symbol by two lines leaving just the circle and the first three levels (horizontal lines). Both symbols work very well, one is not more powerful than the other, they just seem appropriate for different uses/people. Use whichever you feel comfortable with, keep a good intention and they will work wonders! Special symbols like the Master symbol and the "greatest good" work in subtle and powerful ways so the results may take time to become apparent and they might be unexpected!

We can relate the circle at the base of the symbol to the constant cycle of birth, life, and death that all living beings have to experience over and over again, the path to enlightenment being the only exit.

How can we use this symbol and others that we feel are useful? First we have to have faith that the symbol has power to help us. If we don't feel that the symbol is useful to us it won't have a deep impact. We may feel faith in the symbol as soon as we see it and we can deepen our faith by contemplating the benefits of developing our renunciation, compassion, and wisdom.

The main way we can use this symbol is as a connection to the greatest good, to help our relationship become clearer and deeper, and as a transformational tool to help us gradually reduce negative states of mind and develop qualities more "in line" with the greatest good. Remember the symbol is only a key and external manifestation of what we are trying to develop internally. We are not worshiping or venerating an external object simply trying to develop our own greatest good from within. We become like those we associate with; if we hang around with enlightened beings we are very likely to become one eventually! If this symbol can help us develop closer relationships with such energy this is wonderful.

We can use the symbol just on its own or in conjunction with the other Reiki symbols. We can empower it with two power symbols, spend time studying it, incorporating it into artwork, look at it before we fall asleep at night, and generally use our imagination to make the most of its special qualities, or the qualities it represents.

Mainly the "greatest good" is just a symbol that is clear, easy to work with, powerful, and represents something very pure and peaceful. It is not an official Reiki symbol so I am not recommending that we include it in Reiki attunements. Although perhaps we can do this if someone is already attuned; obviously the recipient needs to feel comfortable and close to the symbol and know its origin. I am reluctant to change anything in the attunement process unless I am sure it feels right and mainly prefer to keep everything as close to Dr. Usui's original intention as possible.

Finally, on a practical note, whenever we set a Reiki intention and qualify it for the greatest good that is the best time to use this symbol, we just tag it on the end and let it work for us. To create and activate the greatest good first we need to draw it mentally or physically and say its name three times. We can put it between two power symbols if that feels best although it also seems to work fine on its own and we don't need to be worried about keeping it secret. In fact I feel that the more people who see it the better, I think anyone can use it with a good intention and get excellent results so don't be worried about sharing it with others. Although we need to respect the symbol and perhaps only share it with those whom we feel would appreciate and value it.

I have explained the symbol from a Buddhist perspective but we do not have to accept this explanation to benefit from it. Just regarding it as a representation of the greatest good, like the Master symbol, is enough. We all come from different spiritual/religious backgrounds but the purest aspect of all religions and paths to inner peace are the same and it is this pure nature that is represented by this special symbol.

9

The benefits of regular meditation are now well known. We gain improved health and well-being in many ways, levels of stress are greatly reduced and positive, peaceful, and confident states of mind are easily generated. There are many different types of meditation, most of them aim to relax the body and mind and promote peaceful and positive states of mind. Meditation is a very simple, natural, and powerful way of realizing our abilities to become more whole, healthy, and happy human beings from within. Meditation is not difficult and it does not take years to master. We can receive great benefit even from our very first meditation session. To gain the most from meditation we really need to find a local meditation group that is led by an experienced teacher from an authentic tradition. However, this chapter is designed to give the reader an introduction to meditation and if we follow the instructions carefully we can gain great benefit from practicing for just 10–15 minutes per day.

Relaxation meditation

This can be done either sitting up or lying down. Relaxing music may help and you will need fifteen or twenty minutes of free time.

Begin by making a conscious intention to completely relax your body and mind and receive whatever healing you need during the time you have available for your greatest good. Take some deep breaths and settle into a comfortable position. Try to let go of anything that might be on your mind; this is your time to relax properly and it's important that nothing distracts you.

Bring your attention to your toes and try to "find" any tension and release it. At first it may be helpful to tense and then release them as we need to gradually familiarize ourselves with the experience of consciously relaxing, then the process will become easier. Move your attention slowly into the rest of your feet, consciously relaxing each part. If it helps you can think "release and relax" as you slowly bring your attention to the ankles, shins, calves, knees, etc. Continue to move your attention up through the body, consciously relaxing each part. If your attention wanders, simply return to where you were up to. When you have reached the top of your head spend a few minutes being aware of how it feels to be completely relaxed. The more we remember this experience the easier it will become to repeat and carry it forward into our daily activities. This technique can take some time to master so don't be disappointed if you still feel some tension after the first few sessions; this will pass in time and the technique will become natural. At this point we can stop, dedicate our positive energy, and get up slowly, or we can continue with a simple visualization.

Healing visualization

Visualize a spiraling stream of golden or white light entering through the crown of your head and filling every part of your body, again try to move the light slowly down so you get a sensation that each part of your body and every cell is filled with "light" energy. We can then imagine that our whole body and mind melt into this light, which slowly expands to fill the room, the house, town and country, the whole planet and finally the whole of space. Then spend some time enjoying this experience of pure light filling the whole of space.

If we wish this is a good point to think of others who may need healing, local or world conflicts, disasters, or simply "every living being." Visualize these people or situations surrounded by the light and imagine that all their problems or sickness are easily transformed and healed, then just continue to visualize them as healthy, happy, and content for a few minutes. We can think, "how wonderful, these people are now actually free from their pain and problems," try to really believe that this has happened. Then concentrate for as long as possible on the feeling of joy that arises from this thought.

Don't worry if at first this feels false or manufactured; with sincere, regular practice your motivation will become more natural and powerful. Also don't try too hard or make your visualizations too complicated, an honest intention and a strong belief that your positive thoughts have really helped is the most important aspect.

The power of the mind is limitless, by strongly imagining that through our actions people are released from their problems, this creates the causes for it to actually happen in the future. When you have finished, visualize the light coming slowly back into the space of your body and seal it in with a mental intention like:

Balanced, centered, grounded, blessed, and protected

or something similar or simpler! Then get up slowly when you are ready and dedicate the positive energy you have created. Sometimes when we are setting intentions like the one above or dedicating the positive energy created through a Reiki action, it may be helpful to say or think the intention three times. This sets the intention firmly in our minds and helps us to see if the intention sounds or feel "right," it may be too complicated or not clear enough. We can change an intention simply by saying or thinking a new one that applies to the same person or situation, this will automatically override the previous one, if it is for the "greatest good"! The power of our intentions and dedications are dependent upon the sincerity and stability of our true heartfelt wishes. So we need to keep an eye on them and check them regularly!

Meditation for developing compassion

We prepare for this type of meditation by finding a regular daily quiet time, about fifteen to twenty minutes or more. Early morning is often best when we are fresh and this can really help us start and continue the day in a positive way. The room we use should be peaceful and clean and if we have a particular religious belief we can set up a small shrine or altar with holy pictures, scriptures, and offerings. This serves as a spiritual focal point and helps to build and hold a good quality of energy in the room and house, which is symbolic of our own body and mind. Also if we intentionally honor, clean, and look after this space regularly and treat it with respect, we are definitely creating the causes for our meditations to gradually become clearer and deeper, with long lasting benefits. By inviting the universal blessings or "greatest good" into our house and life, by creating a small shrine, we may also notice many positive benefits in other areas of our life. Also other people may comment that our house always seems peaceful and welcoming!

We can meditate sitting up in a chair with our back straight, but not tense, our feet flat on the floor, and hands resting in our lap, or we can sit on a floor cushion in a traditional meditation posture. In this meditation we relax the body and focus the mind by slowly mentally scanning the body for tension and releasing it, we begin at the top of the head and slowly work down through the various parts of the body until we reach the toes. Then we bring our attention to our breathing and particularly to the sensation at the tip of the nostrils as we feel the cool air coming in and the warm air as we breathe out. We focus on this sensation completely. Our breathing is the "object" of meditation. This focuses the mind and improves our clarity and concentration, in fact this simple breathing meditation, if practiced for ten or fifteen minutes daily, can greatly improve our quality of life by giving us a clear and peaceful mind. If we "lose" our object of meditation and begin thinking about other things, then when we realize this we simply bring our attention back to the sensations of breathing. If we have no experience of meditation it can be helpful to practice just the breathing meditation for several days or weeks before trying anything else.

There are two parts to the next stage of meditation; these are contemplation and placement. Contemplation is the mental process of considering the benefits of abandoning negative thoughts and actions and of adopting positive ones. When, as a result of this reasoning, a strong wish arises in the mind to change our behavior for the better, then this is our object of placement and we "hold it" or experience it for as long as possible.

To develop compassion we can first contemplate how the opposite of compassion – anger/hatred – causes so many problems in the world. In fact as mentioned earlier in this book the selfish mind of anger is responsible for all conflicts and wars. If no one ever experienced anger we would live in a very peaceful world.

We contemplate how angry or selfish thoughts and feelings have caused us many problems and great unhappiness in the past and we consider how wonderful it would be to be free from these heavy negative minds. Then when we naturally feel a strong wish to release these feelings and develop the opposing positive qualities we try to stay with and encourage these positive intentions.

We then contemplate the problems that others experience in their lives. We can think about people we know who are very unhappy or we can think about situations we have heard about or seen on TV where people or animals are suffering. When a feeling of compassion arises in the mind toward these beings we hold onto it for as long as possible and try to mix our mind with it completely, almost as if we have become compassion and that is our nature. Then we make a firm determination or commitment to ourselves to act to help others whenever and in whatever way we can. This determination is the final goal of our meditation and we should try to make it as deep and heartfelt as possible and try to remember that determination throughout the rest of the day.

The key to successful meditation is to consistently make a strong inner determination to let go of negative and damaging ways of living and being and develop more positive harmonious and constructive ones.

If our mind wanders during meditation we simply return to the contemplation until that strong wish to develop our good qualities arises again, then stay with that determination. We are actually training or encouraging ourselves to eventually think and feel this way quite naturally. When we "hold" an object of meditation we should not strain the mind, it should feel natural, as if our mind has completely mixed or become "one" with the object of meditation, i.e. our wish to be more tolerant, patient, or compassionate. By regularly developing these deep wishes to change for the better we will definitely become more positive, happy, content, and considerate.

This ancient tried and tested way of dealing with life's problems, if practiced correctly and regularly, is a guaranteed solution and unlike other modern methods of finding happiness, addiction to it produces very healthy results!

The meditations will also be most effective if we apply them directly to our own lives based on our own life experience. There is no point meditating every day on a vague wish to love others if in our hearts we are not really interested in changing or if these meditations are not directly relevant to our lives. It is possible to use the technique of meditation in this way to actually suppress or avoid our most relevant personal problems, thereby actually deepening these problems and this is of course not meditation!

We have to mentally make the meditations come alive and then carry our good intentions forward into the rest of the day. We do this by remembering the positive feelings and determination that arose during our meditation and trying to use this motivation to guide all our actions of body and mind. Whenever we become aware that negative feelings or thoughts, like worry or impatience, are about to arise in the mind we can prevent them influencing us by recalling our earlier good intentions. In this way our wisdom and happiness will gradually increase and our daily problems will steadily decrease.

Meditiation for developing inner peace

You may find it helpful to try this practice whilst sitting up in a chair, as it is easy to fall asleep when lying down; also begin this practice by doing the breathing meditation explained previously. This calms and stabilizes the mind.

The process of watching the mind or developing mindfulness is also a very powerful way of developing inner peace and the natural intuitive wisdom that brings. Simply look for the moments of natural peace and stay with them. When distractions arise in the mind/body or you are disturbed by a noise don't worry or become irritated/involved, simply "witness" or watch these small events and allow them to come and go, continue watching/experiencing your mind/body and the peace will return sooner or later. Then just follow this inner peace and try to naturally stay with it without straining the mind, so that you become more and more familiar with it. In time this experience will arise more easily and naturally, you will not need to consciously find or stay with it. Eventually this natural inner peace will become your normal state of mind and as you continue this practice you will gain deeper and more profound levels of self-awareness and happiness.

Outdoor healing meditation

This is a very simple and enjoyable meditation to do and it is especially effective if you can do it outside, perhaps in a garden or in the countryside. You can use a tree to rest your back against whilst you are doing it, as trees can act as a gateway or junction for the energy exchange.

There is a natural exchange of life force energy between a tree, the earth, and the universe and it is this exchange that you need to become aware of and part of. In some oriental philosophies trees are seen as symbolic or actual gateways between heaven and earth, with their roots soaking up nutrients from the earth and their leaves stretching toward the light of the sun and the energy that it gives. Indeed Buddha attained enlightenment whilst seated in meditation beneath a great tree, the Bodhi tree. Trees are also seen as an example of how we should approach life. Growing steadily year by year a tree is strong yet balanced and able to change with the seasons, it bends and does not break in high winds because its roots are deep, it is flexible and adaptable to the forces of nature. When the conditions are right, as in summer, its growth rate increases accordingly and in winter it rests and recharges. Likewise we can only be effective spiritual beings if our feet are firmly planted on the ground and we know when it is time to challenge ourselves and time to rest.

Choose a tree that you feel drawn to and place your back against it, with your feet or backside between two roots if they are showing above ground. Take a few moments to get comfortable and "tune in" to your surroundings, then close your eyes and slowly relax your body and mind. Set an "intent" to receive and give healing energy for your and others' "greatest good." Then once you have taken your remedy imagine white or golden light spiraling through your crown chakra (the top of your head) and filling your body and mind until you feel completely peaceful and relaxed. Then visualize this light entering the earth through your base chakra or feet and descending directly to the center of the planet. From there the energy radiates throughout the whole planet, touching all humans and animals, surrounding all the towns and cities, then out through our solar system to the whole universe and all worlds and realms of existence, seen and unseen. We strongly believe that all living beings are released from their problems and blessed with this healing energy, the nature of love, compassion, and wisdom. Then the main emphasis of this practice is to concentrate on the feeling of joy that arises from believing that we have directly helped others. Try to let your mind merge with an ocean of loving joy. You can stay with this experience for as long as you wish before slowly bringing your attention back to where you are sitting. This universal healing is a very powerful and compassionate act. When you have finished, as always, you can dedicate your good karma and if you wish protect your own energy system by thinking and feeling:

I am fully blessed and protected.

Mantra meditation

A mantra is a special word or group of words that when spoken or thought have a positive effect on the mind and body. There are many mantras used in Buddhism to heal, purify, and help us develop certain positive qualities of mind. The word mantra means "mind protection." Mantra appears to us as words or sound, although the Buddhist Sutras or Holy Scriptures tell us that in reality mantra is life force energy.

One of the most well known mantras is OM MANE PADME HUM, roughly translated these Sanskrit letters mean "all praise to the jewel in the lotus" although they have deep meaning on many levels. The "jewel in the lotus" refers to our Buddha nature or greatest potential for good; this arises from the lotus, which is the symbol of compassion. So we can see that the mind of compassion or the wish to develop compassion is the source of our greatest potential and is worth the highest "praise."

OM MANE PADME HUM is the mantra of compassion and has a profound effect on the heart chakra, it brings great inner peace and contentment. We can use this mantra at any time as mentioned above or we can receive a special empowerment from a Buddhist Geshe or Master and combine the mantra with an especially powerful but simple form of meditation practice to develop our compassion and ripen our potential for benefiting others. For this mantra we would need the empowerment of Buddha Avalokiteshvara, the Buddha of Compassion. Buddha Avalokiteshvara had such a great wish to help others that he blessed his own name so that when anyone said it three times they would receive relief from fear. This is still a very effective way to prevent and relieve fear.

There are many ways we can use mantra meditations to heal ourselves and others. If our intentions are truly compassionate this is an especially powerful action or karma as the nature of mantra is so pure, holy, and blessed. We can say mantras for others whenever they need help, perhaps for people who are distressed, sick, and homeless, even for dying animals or insects, this will help them greatly. Then we can also dedicate the future effects of our actions or karma for their benefit. This is a special form of "giving" and will also greatly increase the power of the karma that returns to us in the future.

To develop our wisdom we would need to receive the empowerment and use the mantra of Buddha Manjushri, the Wisdom Buddha. To develop our healing abilities we would need to receive the empowerment of Medicine Buddha (Sange Menhla in Tibetan), the embodiment of all the Buddha's healing qualities.

If we want to practice or know more about the different types of mantra meditations we need to study appropriate texts or receive teachings from a qualified and experienced teacher.

Toward true wisdom

One of the special qualities of authentic meditation is that it increases our wisdom. Wisdom is very different from intellectual ability. Many intelligent people are very unhappy. Since all living beings have the same basic wish to avoid problems and find happiness, wisdom is simply the ability to understand where lasting happiness comes from. As we meditate daily we will come to see that happiness is simply a state of mind and that since we have the opportunity to create positive states of mind through meditation, prayer, etc., these methods are the key to lasting happiness. Although the essence and practice of meditation is quite simple, as mentioned it is a good idea to seek out a fully qualified and experienced teacher who can guide us along the stages of the path of meditation. If we try to learn on our own or from a book we may encounter many problems and waste much time and consequently we can lose interest because we are not experiencing consistently good results. Learning and sharing our experiences with others, meditating in a group and having the opportunity to ask questions can greatly assist our enjoyment and progress. Also, having a teacher who is a living example of what we can achieve through meditation is a constant inspiration and encouragement to our own developing practice.

If we do a little meditation every day good results will accumulate, we shall become more relaxed and more able to enjoy life fully; gradually we shall become a true source of wisdom, compassion, and inner strength. (For more information on meditation see Appendix 4 and 5.)

10

─THE FINAL RESULT─

Pure and simple

There is definitely a great need for Reiki in this world. We are living in times of great change, transformation, and opportunity. The world has changed so much in recent decades, and no doubt will continue along this path for some time to come. As individuals we have a responsibility to take a positive role in this opportunity for spiritual awakening and inner transformation.

Our actions, our decisions, even our thoughts and feelings have an effect on the world around us. If one person in a family allows themselves to become negative and pessimistic we know that this has a negative effect on the whole family. If a family has a generally negative approach to life we know this can have an adverse effect on a whole street or community. If one nation has a sense of superiority over another we can say that this attitude affects the whole world.

As individuals our approach to life can have a direct effect on our friends and family, this in turn has an effect on our community, our nation, and our whole world. If we want to have a positive effect on the whole world first we need to feel that the happiness of others is important. At the moment we tend to feel that our own happiness and that of our family and friends is most important and we tend not to consider the welfare of others. One of the best things we can do for our world is to develop a mind that feels a deep concern for others, those in our local community, our nation, and the whole world.

We could take this as our main spiritual aim or intention. We do not need to be physically close to others to feel close to them. All we need to do is to regularly try to develop a compassionate feeling or attitude toward others wherever they may be and in time this will become our natural state of mind. It will take time and effort but the quality of such an inner transformation is well worth it. By doing this we are putting ourselves in line or in tune with the greatest good and this helps to receive and channel a more subtle or profound level of Reiki.

As practitioners of higher Reiki one of the main benefits of developing a mind that cherishes all living beings is that we show a good example to other Reiki and non-Reiki people. The more people who develop a spiritually mature, responsible, and compassionate approach to life the more our world will become a beautiful place to live. If many people are holding the whole world in their hearts the future is bright.

—APPENDIX 1—

OM AH HUM meditation

Although the OM AH HUM mantra is very short it is one of the most blessed mantras, it represents or is an expression of the body, speech and mind of all the Buddhas. It is very helpful if we can remember this whilst we are doing the meditation and especially develop the wish to transform our own body, speech and mind in that of an enlightened being for the benefit of others.

Developing this motivation before we begin to meditate is very important, it will make our meditation more powerful and we create the karma to become an enlightened being in the future.

Intention is everything. If we live our lives with the intention to find happiness for ourselves this is quite a narrow mind, considering how many living beings there are, who all wish to be happy. If we can learn to focus on the welfare of others more than our own this shows great wisdom, as this is the mind that will in fact bring us most happiness, but most importantly it will bring peace to the world and have a very positive influence on others.

In this meditation we combine breathing meditation and mantra recitation. As with all meditation we need to find a peaceful environment and sit comfortably with our back fairly straight but not too straight and our hands resting gently in our lap.

Breathe naturally through the nostrils and spend some time mentally checking through the body from head to foot to see if you can find any tension. Allow your self to fully relax and simply imagine any tension draining away down through the body and into the floor. When you are fully relaxed bring you attention to your breathing, becoming aware of the natural rise and fall of the breath.

To develop some clarity in the mind we can try to focus on the gentle sensation at the tip of the nostrils as the cool air comes in and the warm air goes out. We can do this for maybe five minutes, if we find that we have been distracted we simply bring our attention back to our 'object' of meditation.

When our mind is relaxed and focused we can begin to mentally recite the OM AH HUM mantra. As we inhale we mentally recite OM, then we hold our breath at our heart for a short time and recite AH, them we exhale and recite HUM at the same time. We repeat this process for as long as we wish.

This very simple meditation brings profound results. If we practice for 10–15 minutes everyday, in time our mind will become more and more peaceful and less distracted. In time we will find it difficult to become agitated, unpeaceful, or angry. Inner peace will become our natural state of mind and we will gradually draw closer and closer to full enlightenment.

The Reiki crystal method

A crystal formation can be created and charged with Reiki which will constantly send Reiki for healing purposes (or to achieve a positive intention/wish) for days or weeks after it has been created.

To create the crystal formation you will need at least seven clear quartz points and another larger than the rest or a crystal pyramid. Select ones that you feel have a clear and powerful vibration or energy. You can clean the crystals by holding them under cold running water and leaving them in a place where the morning sun can charge them every morning for a few days, for example on a window ledge or actually outside on a lawn. Some people like to cleanse crystals by leaving them in sea salt water for a day or actually bury them in the Earth. Also spend some time charging/cleansing each crystal with Reiki and the power symbol, especially the central one.

Select a good place for your crystal formation, it should be clean and quiet so that it will not be disturbed, or as near to this as possible. Place the largest crystal or pyramid in the center and the other crystals around and pointing toward it in a circle about 15cm away (or whatever feels right to you).

Find a photograph of yourself which you feel is 'honest' and write your name on the back. Also draw the four Reiki symbols on the back along with their names. Think about a good intention, which may be specific or general such as "May I receive whatever I need for the greatest good." Repeat this for other people or situations you would like to send Reiki to. If you do not have a photograph just write their name or an appropriate title on a piece of paper.

Place the photo or piece of paper under the central crystal face up, it might feel appropriate to charge each crystal again (including a power symbol) and place it back in its position in the formation. Charge the main crystal last and while it is in your hand think about your intention again. Before you place it in the center of the circle draw all four the Reiki symbols over it. Place it in the center and put both hands over the center of the crystal formation palms down, so you can charge the grid with Reiki. After a few minutes set your intention and draw the symbols over the center of the formation as you would for a sending an absentee treatment. It can help if your intention includes the wish for the people or situations to receive constant Reiki until the difficulty is resolved. Then to finish again hold you palms over the grid for three minutes, each minute represents four of the twelve Reiki positions in a full treatment. If it feels right you can recharge the central crystal for a few minutes each day. You can add and remove photos and intentions on a daily basis again each time you do this recharge the main crystal and every few weeks dismantle, cleanse and recreate the whole formation.

APPENDIX 3

Reiki organizations

The Reiki Alliance,
PO Box 41,
Cataldo,
ID83810,
USA.
TEL: 1 208 682 3535.
FAX: 1 208 682 4848.
E-MAIL: 75051.3471@compuserve.com

The Reiki Alliance,
Postbus 75523 1070 AM,
Amsterdam,
Netherlands.
TEL: 31 20 6719276.
FAX: 31 20 6711736.
E-MAIL: 100125.466@compuserve.com

The Reiki Alliance,
Cornbrook Bridge House,
Clee Hill,
Ludlow,
Shropshire,
SY8 3QQ.
TEL/FAX: 01584 891197.
E-MAIL: KateReikiJones@compuserve.com

UK Reiki Federation,
PO BOX 1785,
Andover,
Hampshire.
TEL: 01264 773774.
E-MAIL: enquiry@reikifed.co.uk
WEBSITE: www.reikifed.co.uk

Meditation classes near you

The demand for a lasting solution to the problems of stress and anxiety, created by the nature of today's 'material' society, has led to the setting up of meditation groups in almost every town and city. These groups vary in content and in their spiritual origin, so it is important to find one that you feel comfortable with, one that is run by a fully qualified teacher and one that teaches a recognized and correct 'path' true to the origins of meditation.

Buddhist meditation

Most meditation groups can trace their origins back to Buddha, who lived over 2000 years ago. He was born into one of the richest and most powerful royal families in India and spent the first twenty-nine years of his life living as a prince. However despite having all the health, wealth and good relationships he could wish for he still felt incomplete and he could also see a great need in others for a real solution to life's problems. Finally he came to understand that most people look for happiness in the wrong place! He felt sure that true, lasting, happiness could be found simply by understanding and developing the mind. He decided to give up his inheritance and devote the rest of his life to attaining the ultimate state of wisdom and happiness, so that he could share this with others. All Buddha's teachings were recorded and passed down and to this day we have a pure, unbroken lineage of the path to full enlightenment. This lineage is now firmly established in the West. We do not have to travel far to find it!

New kadampa tradition

One of the largest international Buddhist organizations is the New Kadampa Tradition. Established in 1976 by Tibetan meditation master, Geshe Kelsang Gyatso Rinpoche. Its purpose is "to present the mainstream of Buddhist teachings in a way that is relevant and immediately applicable to the contemporary Western way of life." Most cities and towns in the U.K. have an NKT residential center or meditation group and many others are opening in the U.S.A, Europe and all over the world (see Appendix 5 for books by Geshe Kelsang Gyatso on Buddhism and Meditation). To find your nearest Buddhist center or if you would like a teacher to give an introductory talk on Buddhism in your area please contact:

Main Contact:

NEW KADAMPA TRADITION,
Conishead Priory,
Ulverston,
Cumbria,
ENGLAND,
LA12 9QQ
TEL/FAX: 01229 588533 (within UK).
E-MAIL: kadampa@dircon.co.uk
WEBSITE: www.kadampa.net

U.S.A. Contact:

NEW KADAMPA TRADITION
The Kadampa Meditation Center,
Sweeney Road,
Glen Spey NY 12737, USA.
TEL: (845) 856-9000
TOLL FREE: 1-877-KADAMPA (1-877-523-2672)
FAX: (845) 856-2110
E-MAIL: info@kadampacenter.org

Books on Buddhism

For beginners and more experienced practitioners, the following books are written by Geshe Kelsang Gyatso and published by Tharpa Publications:

Transform Your Life – A Blissful Journey
Introduction to Buddhism – An Explanation of the Buddhist Way of Life
The New Meditation Handbook – A Practical Guide to Meditation
Universal Compassion – Transforming Your Life Through Love and Compassion
Eight Steps to Happiness – Transform Your Mind, Transform Your Life
Joyful Path of Good Fortune – The Complete Buddhist Path to Enlightenment
Meaningful to Behold – The Bodhisattva's Way of Life
Guide to the Bodhisattva's Way of Life – A Buddhist Poem for Today

There are many other more advanced and in depth titles on Buddhism available from Tharpa Publications; they also produce Buddhist art reproductions, tapes, talking books, and books in Braille. For more information visit www.tharpa.com

INDEX